Intermittent Fasting And The Keto Diet

Guide for Cleansing Your Body, Losing Weight, and Living a Healthy Lifestyle

Charlotte Melhoff

liable for any hardship or damages that may befall them after undertaking information described herein.

Additionally, the information in the following pages is intended only for informational purposes and should thus be thought of as universal. As befitting its nature, it is presented without assurance regarding its prolonged validity or interim quality. Trademarks that are mentioned are done without written consent and can in no way be considered an endorsement from the trademark holder.

Table of Contents

Introduction

Congratulations on purchasing my book *Intermittent Fasting and the Keto Diet* and thank you for doing so.

The following chapters will discuss what exactly Intermittent Fasting is and how it can be used in conjunction with the Keto Diet. We talk about the scientific approach to Intermittent Fasting and Ketosis as well as how to incorporate both of them into your life. We give you prime examples of recipes that can be used while on the keto diet and explain why they are ideal recipes for the Intermittent Fasting as well. We explain ketosis and how it happens with a detailed breakdown of every step that goes into ketones and ketosis. We explain how to use Intermittent Fasting for optimal health. We also discuss the schedules that work best with a fasting diet. We talk about studies that have proven the benefits of these two in combination with each other. We discuss whether or not you should participate in this type of diet.

We also have in-depth details on challenges and complications that could arise from the keto diet. We talk about what to expect when staring Intermittent Fasting. We have provided you with a list of acceptable foods to eat as well as foods to avoid. Then we give you a few substitutions for your normal carb intake. We go into detail on why this diet plan can work for you during work and at home, and how exercise can increase your chances of success. We talk about how to build a 1-week meal plan and even give you an example of a 1-week meal plan that works for Intermittent Fasting and the Keto diet. There is so much detail and information in this book that you should have no trouble starting Intermittent Fasting and the Keto Diet.

There are plenty of books on this subject on the market. Thanks again for choosing this one! Every effort was made to ensure it is full of as much useful information as possible. Please enjoy!

Chapter 1:
What Is Intermittent Fasting?

Intermittent Fasting is similar to the calorie restriction diet. However, with Intermittent Fasting, you are limiting your intake of food and drinks to a prespecified amount of time. Many people will spend anywhere from 12 to 48 hours without eating while on a fast. Most of us do not eat from around 9 pm to roughly 9 am so fasting is not much different than what we are already doing. However, in fasting, we will be extending that fasting time period by a few more hours. This sounds like it wouldn't be that difficult, and if you think about it, it probably isn't. The key to Intermittent Fasting is to make sure you are getting proper nutrients during the times that you are not fasting.

Fasting is something that has been around for a while especially in religious culture. However, many people are now fasting for weight loss and healthy lifestyle changes. Intermittent Fasting is best accomplished when you are aware of the feed state and the fasting state. The feed state is when you are supplying your body with nutrients that it needs to sustain life. In this state, it is absorbing, digesting, and assimilating the nutrients from your meals. This is the state at which most of us are at during our typical day. At this point, fat burning isn't our priority.

The fasting state is the time when you would normally be asleep. However, in Intermittent Fasting, you are spending waking hours in a fasting state. This helps you process the fat that you have taken in during the feed state. In this state, you are able to use your ketones for energy. The advantage to doing Keto with the Intermittent Fasting is that you are already restricting carbs and glucose. This means that you aren't changing too much about your normal eating habits. Because of the fasting periods on your Intermittent Fasting diet, you will go into ketosis much quicker. It has also been suggested that doing Intermittent Fasting on the Keto diet can help eliminate symptoms of the Keto flu, which is an asymptomatic condition that can take place when your body is going into ketosis. We will talk more about the keto flu in Chapter 3.

Remember that in general, Intermittent Fasting is a meal-timing tool that helps you control the calories you eat. It is not necessarily a diet plan; however, it shows positive results when used with the Keto diet. Because we are fasting for 16 hours and only eating for 8 hours, we are allowing our body to use the fat that is stored for our energy source, and this helps the body go into ketosis much sooner.

How can you use Intermittent Fasting along with the Keto Diet?

Intermittent Fasting is an absolutely terrific way of limiting your available window for eating without disrupting your entire life. What this means is that you will only eat for a few hours out of your day. You can consume as much as your body will allow in those few hours. Most of the time you usually fast for 12-20 hours. Some have fasted up to 36 hours but no more than 48 hours at a time.

During your fasting window, you should not eat or drink anything that has caloric value. This means that you can drink water, black coffee, or tea that has been sweetened with Stevia or erythritol. However, nothing else should be consumed during your fasting period.

There is a daily number of macronutrients that you need to target during your non-fasting times. You should reach this target without restricting what you eat. Although, you may find yourself not meeting this target. Do not worry. Your body will stop you when it is no longer needing any food. Basically, you need to eat protein in large quantities, keep your carbs low, no more than 30 g net carbs, and use fat as a filler for long-term fullness. The basic concept is to help you break through those stubborn months where you have a plateau in your weight loss efforts and need a boost.

Basic principles of Intermittent Fasting

Intermittent Fasting has all the benefits that you would get from carb restriction without any of the downsides. When you fast, you naturally restrict calories. There is no forcing of calorie restriction; it just comes naturally. The reason is that you will most likely not feel like eating more; instead, you will eat less. For instance, eating a large meal right after you have fasted will not cause any excess fat. When you normally overeat, you would have excess fat. Instead, it just makes up for the time period where you ate very little.

When you use fasting, along with your low-carb diet, your body is going to use the fat that is stored up for energy. This will result in a loss of body fat. Since we are doing Intermittent Fasting with The Keto Diet, we are using our fat and ketones for energy, and we are no longer using glucose for our energy. This is helping us lose weight and have control of our appetite, allowing us to stay fuller for a much longer period of time.

Intermittent Fast And The Keto Diet

There are a few different types of Intermittent Fasting that can be done for optimum health and weight loss.

One way to use Intermittent Fasting with the Keto Diet is to skip a meal every now and then. This should be done gradually over time without forcing the fasting. The goal is not to feel hunger. How you can slowly start this process is to extend the time between meals each day. For instance, start by not eating breakfast first thing in the morning for 4-5 days. The next week, go for two more hours before eating breakfast on those same days. The week after that, skip breakfast all together on those same days. This will gradually work fasting into your schedule by skipping a meal 4-5 times a week. You can make your schedule however you like it whether you skip breakfast Monday through Friday or every other day. Maybe you even skip breakfast for 2 days and eat breakfast for 1. Whichever helps you with your Intermittent Fasting is up to you. Oftentimes, people will not fast on the weekends and eat breakfast then.

Most Keto dieters will eat only when hungry. They understand that they are eating high-fat, moderate protein and low-carb foods so this allows them to listen for when they are hungry and eat at those times.

Another approach to Intermittent Fasting with the Keto Diet is to take a 24-hour break and break it into two segmented windows. This would be the 16/8 diet plan. What 16/8 stands for is that you are only fasting for 16 hours. During this time period, you only drink water or tea. During the 8-hour time period, you are eating the calories that you need to sustain life. 16/8 is not the only way to break this down. You can do 20/4 and even 21/3. Whatever works best for you is most important.

If you are a very active person who loves exercise, then try Intermittent Fasting with the Keto diet for exercise. This adds extra calories for boosting your energy. It is similar in details to the previous style of fasting. However, you will incorporate exercise into the schedule. Exercise is good for your body and maintaining weight loss. You will want to hold off on exercise during your fasting period. What you want to do is eat the bulk of your nutrients and macronutrients directly after you exercise. When including exercise into your diet plan, you want to make sure your macronutrients are in line with your goals whether it is muscle gain, fat loss, or body composition. Basically, the days you work out should have more carbs consumed, and then the days you rest, you should eat more fat. Your protein should be high for all days. Make sure your feeding window is the same on every day. That way, you are consistent and can easily stick with your plan. This type of fasting can take a bit of time to schedule out and adjust your lifestyle around. Due to the variations in the meal scheduling, you should plan a meal prep schedule along with a workout schedule that works with your current commitments.

Alternating days of fasting with days that you are unrestricted is another great way to incorporate Intermittent Fasting into your keto lifestyle. Because this is more extreme, it is not advised for everyone. You should start with one of the above methods before jumping into the alternating-days approach. It is best to only include 1 or 2 days of fasting in the week. On these days, you will restrict all intake of food or drinks that have caloric value.

Another alternative to alternate fasting is to alternate days of calorie restriction with days of unrestrictive eating, making sure your meals go along with the keto diet. This approach to Intermittent Fasting can be easier to adjust to since it is not a complete day of fasting. Basically, you will reduce your calorie intake by about 20-30% on one day, and then the next day, you will eat anything within the original keto diet guidelines.

Lastly, combining the fat fasting with Intermittent fasting along with keto is another great way to include this in your diet approach. Where you would normally eat 5 small meals on a traditional fat fast, on this approach, you will eat 1 to 2 regular high-fat meals which makes things much easier for someone just starting out with this fasting approach to dieting.

The key takeaway is that whatever approach you take doesn't matter as long as it works for you and your lifestyle. Do what works for you, and it will work out. You should be able to meet your macronutrients goals on most days and remember that Intermittent Fasting is not about starving.

The basic ideas behind Intermittent Fasting with the Keto Diet

The idea behind Intermittent Fasting and the Keto diet is that you are eating a healthy meal with times of fasting that help digest your food and place you into ketosis faster than you would otherwise go into it. While on the keto diet, it is hard to gain muscle mass. However, we combine this with the Intermittent Fasting, which helps with your body's insulin sensitivity, as well as your growth hormone and blood glucose regulation. Due to these benefits, you are able to build muscle mass while doing both of these diets together. Another reason why they work so well together is that while on the keto diet, you are trying to reach ketosis. With Intermittent Fasting being used in combination, you can reach ketosis much faster. Intermittent Fasting helps you reach ketosis faster due to the change in your metabolism that it brings about. It keeps your metabolism in a high state, which quickly adapts you to the lower carb intake.

After reaching ketosis, you are able to sustain the Intermittent Fasting much easier because you will no longer experience the hunger cramps. While fasting, your body is using the fat from the energy you have at this time, and this leads to a lower body fat percentage and in the long run, a leaner body.

What exactly is Ketosis?

Ketosis is the body's way of using fat that is stored as energy. Normally, our bodies use the carbs that we take in as our energy source. This is stored in two ways. Glycogenesis is the process where excess glucose is converted to glycogen. Glycogen is the body's form of stored sugar. It is stored in the liver and in the muscles. Generally, these levels are depleted in 6-24 hours based on the person's body size, activity, and so on.

The second way of storing energy is lipogenesis which is our back-up storage system. This is where glucose is turned to fat for storage to be used at a later time. Glycogen stores are limited where fat stores are unlimited. This gives us an extra bit of energy sources for when we run out of our glycogen storage. This is how you would be sustained for weeks and months without adequate nutrients and food. When we start to restrict our carb intake, the glycogenesis and lipogenesis become inactive. So instead the processes of glycogenolysis and lipolysis take over. This frees up energy from the glycogen and fat stores. This is when your body starts processing ketones from your fat instead of the glycogen. Ketones come from the body's breakdown of fat into fatty acid and glycerol.

Yes, we can use the fatty acids and glycerol for an energy source in many of our cells. The brain does not use them at all. Due to the slowness of the process, it is not an optimal support for the function of the brain. That is why our body starts with sugar instead of fat for the energy source.

Ketones are formed by breaking fat down into fatty acids and glycerol, then they are processed through the liver, and at this time, they are converted into sugar and ketones. The glycerol undergoes something called gluconeogenesis, which is the conversion to sugar we talked about earlier. The fatty acids during the process called ketogenesis are converted to ketones. In this process, the acetoacetate is produced.

This is then converted to two other forms of ketones.

- Beta-hydroxybutyrate or BHB, which is a much more efficient source of energy fuel, can take place a couple of weeks after you have reached ketosis. This undergoes extra chemical reactions and makes for a more efficient energy source for the cells. The body and brain prefer to use the BHB and acetoacetate for energy due to it being 70% more efficient.

- Acetone is mostly waste. However, it can also be metabolized into glucose. It is the culprit behind the smelly breath that keto dieters have.

Throughout your time in ketosis, your body will eventually start to expel fewer ketones. By using keto sticks, you can track the process and see the slowdown progression.

What Intermittent Fasting would look like in your life

By incorporating Intermittent Fasting into your life, you will see a difference in when you eat along with what you eat. You will have more energy and less health-related issues. Intermittent Fasting provides you with a period of rest from eating. By using this in your life, you will start to adjust to how much your body really needs of caloric value in a day. This helps you to lose weight. You will also find yourself enjoying food again and wanting to do other things like movement and activity to get healthier because you will start to feel healthier and more active. You will also see a mindset shift where you will think more positively about yourself and be positive about your weight loss goals. This is one reason why Intermittent Fasting is a great option for those who are on the keto diet. It helps to shift the mindset into a more positive and less stressed mindset allowing for optimal goal accomplishment.

Brief Overview of This Chapter

- *We discussed what the intermittent Fasting diet is and some key facts to help you understand how it is done.*

- *Then we discussed how you can use it along with the Keto diet.*

- *Next, we talked about the basic principles behind the Intermittent Fasting and the Keto diet program. How it is accomplished and what it means.*

- *Finally, we discussed how it would look in your life if you were participating in the Intermittent Fasting and the Keto diet.*

Chapter 2:
The Benefits of the Keto diet

The benefits of Intermittent Fasting are similar, if not the same, as restricting calorie intake. However, there is a vast difference in the way the benefits will benefit your body. Intermittent Fasting can improve your metabolic syndrome markers. What this means is that it improves your blood lipids, improves your insulin resistance, increases insulin sensitivity, reduces blood pressure, and inflammation markers as well as cardiovascular markers.

Throughout the scientific studies of Intermittent Fasting, they have noticed a connection between a longer lifespan and fasting. It apparently affects the aging process due to the calorie restriction. This can also be contributed to the improvement of symptoms of metabolic syndromes such as diabetes, obesity, and such. It has also proven that it reduces your risk of cancer.

Your body has its own ability to heal itself, and the process of ketosis has been proven to enhance this ability which is called autophagy. Autophagy is a process by which your body can heal itself, and it is a required process that is used for muscle mass maintenance. It also has several anti-aging properties. Fasting has also been shown to enhance production of your growth hormone. This is something that decreases as we get older. However, with fasting, we can enhance the growth hormone.

There are several metabolic factors that can be strongly linked to cancers of various types. Some of those factors in men are high blood pressure as well as triglycerides. The cancer-causing factor in women is associated with high plasma glucose. Due to its improvements in metabolic syndrome markers, you are reducing your risk of cancer as well as helping with the negative side effects of chemotherapy in patients already diagnosed with cancer.

Studies have been done to determine the benefits of fasting and ketosis for brain function and mental clarity. Once you have reached ketosis, this means you are no longer glucose-dependent. This can take 3 to 4 weeks, and you will be able to start using ketones for energy. This helps reduce your brain fog and provides you with more mental focus and clarity. They have found that patients that use fasting with keto have a higher capacity for learning and enhancing their mental clarity. Studies on fasting with keto have shown improvement in neurodegenerative diseases such as Alzheimer's, Huntington's disease, Parkinson's disease, and stroke. They also found that there was an increase in the resistance of neurons in the brain which lowers the dysfunction and degeneration of the neurons.

As scientific research advances and continues to learn more about fasting with the keto diet, more areas of study have been performed to include fitness, weight loss, and many other health benefits. During a fasting state, your exercise can enhance your fat burning, allowing for more fat consumption for energy usage. Fasting has been shown to have a positive effect on performance in those who exercise regularly while fasting. There are two different studies for fasting with exercise. One of the studies shows an increased performance level while the other one shows no additional benefits to fasting and exercise combined. They have also found that fasting while exercising does not decrease muscle tone, but instead, it enhances your recovery after exercise and muscle protein synthesis.

The weight loss benefits are just as impressive as the health benefits we have already listed above. With fasting, you eat the same amount of food that you would normally eat. However, you eat all your nutrient-rich foods in a smaller time period allowing you to fast throughout the week. This, by itself, is not the reason for weight loss in participants of the Intermittent Fasting and Keto diet plan. Instead of being the defining factor in weight loss, it simply helps the participants to eat less caloric value which enhances their weight loss goals. The key concept is that once you are keto adapted, your body will require less food intake, and if you are eating 2 large meals instead of 3 regular meals, then your intake is decreased, allowing you to eat less and lose weight.

Another benefit that has been connected to Intermittent Fasting with the Keto diet is fat oxidation. The increase of growth hormone and a decrease of insulin levels combined help us lose body fat. Since Intermittent Fasting is less restrictive than a calorie restrictive diet, many people are turning to fasting for their health and weight loss goals.

The science behind the Keto Diet

The Keto diet is a low-carb, moderate protein, and high-fat eating plan, that when used in the right way, it can place the body into a state of ketosis. Ketosis is what happens when your body starts using ketones from the liver as an energy source. Ketones are the broken-down processed fats that have been filtered through the liver.

The science behind the Keto diet is explained with the understanding of how the body works and produces energy. In order for us to have energy, we have to eat carbs and fat. The carbs and fat are broken down into an energy source and then our body utilizes it as needed. Energy is produced by processing carbs into glucose and insulin and processing fat into ketones.

Why Intermittent Fasting and the Keto diet work well together

Intermittent Fasting and Keto work well together because they balance each other out. With keto, you are working towards a weight loss goal by burning fat for energy instead of carbs. Keto helps to place your body into ketosis which is a way of manipulating your metabolism into using the fat that is stored in your body as your energy source instead of the glucose. A diet high in fat will take longer for your body to digest which gives you a more satisfied feeling for longer than when you eat carbs or protein. This satiated feeling also lowers your snack cravings, allowing you to lower your caloric intake per day.

By lowering your carbs, you are lowering your blood sugar which helps balance your insulin needs. This diet has been shown to improve your sensitivity to insulin which is a crucial part of weight loss. Stabilizing your blood sugar has helped many people eliminate brain fog and improve focus, memory, and concentration. The combination of keto and fasting has also shown great improvements in those that have Type 2 diabetes. The key factor in using Intermittent Fasting and Keto together is that while doing Keto you can kick-start your ketosis so that you can reach your goals sooner.

Who should not be using the Keto diet?

- Type 1 diabetics should not be using the Intermittent Fasting and keto diet. When you fast, it causes your blood sugar to drop; this can be problematic for those suffering from Type 1 Diabetes. When the blood sugar drops, it can cause hypoglycemia. If you are on insulin or insulin- lowering drugs, then you should definitely check with your doctor about whether or not the Intermittent Fasting and keto diet is okay for you. Sometimes, you can speak with your doctor, and they will lower your insulin shots or medication so that you can use Intermittent Fasting and keto diet to get healthy.

- People who suffer from adrenal and thyroid issues should approach the Intermittent Fasting and keto diet with caution. Those that suffer from these issues are not good at handling stress in their bodies so this could be more problematic than helpful. Fasting can cause stress on the body, and this could exacerbate their conditions.

- If you are suffering from an eating disorder, you might find that fasting is not the right way to maintain your weight. Intermittent Fasting can exacerbate your disorder and make it difficult for you to get healthy. However, you should completely avoid long-term fasting. If you wish to try Intermittent Fasting, you should definitely consult a doctor.

- Children are not a good fit for the Intermittent Fasting and keto diet. Due to the fact that they are still growing and need adequate nutrition daily, this should not be tried by anyone under the age of 18.

- People who are underweight and undernourished should not try Intermittent Fasting and the keto diet. If your BMI is 18 kg/m2 or less, it is not recommended to fast at all. This can cause a malnourishment that will eventually make them unhealthier and could possibly kill them.

- Pregnant or breastfeeding moms should not use the Intermittent Fasting and keto diet. While breastfeeding, you need to have all the nutrients you can. Limiting your food intake or fasting would cause undue harm to yourself and your baby.

Brief Overview of This Chapter

- *In this chapter, we discussed the benefits of being on the keto diet along with intermittent Fasting and how it can improve your health.*

- *We also discussed the changes it makes in your body and how that enhances your weight loss and increases your healthy immunity.*

- *Then we discussed the science behind Intermittent Fasting and how it has been studied for years to find the effectiveness of it in conjunction with the Keto diet.*

- *Lastly, we discussed why Intermittent Fasting and the Keto diet work together so well and how they complement each other and enhance the results for each goal.*

Chapter 3:
Challenges that You May Face with Intermittent Fasting and the Keto Diet

Oftentimes, we do not consider the challenges that we will face when starting something new. With the Intermittent Fasting and Keto diet, there are several challenges that we have to consider. Everything comes with challenges. It is knowing how to alleviate or avoid those challenges that makes trying new things easier and safer for us.

Constipation

Constipation is a big challenge that many people face while on the Keto diet. Due to the reduction in carbs and fiber, you may find that you are more constipated than normal. This can be because of increased digestive issues. However, you can fix this with lots of water, some digestive enzymes, some leafy greens, and high-fiber vegetables. You can also increase your avocado intake to help alleviate these symptoms. When you supplement with a digestive enzyme, make sure it contains lipase, which is the primary enzyme that breaks down dietary fats. This will also help with the avocado and olive oil that you are likely adding to your daily diet.

Dehydration

Dehydration can be one of the more serious challenges you will face when trying the Keto diet. Due to cutting back on carbs, your body will produce less insulin. This decreases your glycogen stores. When we take in carbs, we place them in storage for use as an energy source. When we store our carbs or glycogen, we are also storing 3 g of water. By reducing our carb intake, we are depleting those stores, which causes our kidneys to excrete more water. This, in turn, helps us to reduce water weight. However, this weight loss is short-lived. You will feel less bloated, which makes you look better. The downside is that when you flush your water resources, then you are losing minerals called electrolytes. Electrolytes are important for muscle contractions, body temperature, heartbeat regulation, bladder control, neurological functions, and energy production. Simply put, without electrolytes, you would not be alive.

Jagged weight loss or plateaued weight loss

With every new thing in our life, we will experience ups and downs that make us feel like we are not succeeding. However, with the Intermittent Fasting and Keto diet, you are going to have to trust that it is working and avoid checking your weight for a while. Once you gradually start to see changes, consider checking your weight loss on the scale. Do not be discouraged. Every weight loss plan has a period of ups and downs as well as plateaus.

Low Energy

During the metabolic transition that will produce ketones for your energy source, you will probably experience fatigue, brain fog, and weakness. This is normal. However, make sure you are getting the essential nutrients including electrolytes. Making sure you are not dehydrated can alleviate these symptoms. Oftentimes, adding some bone broth to your daily fluid intake can help add electrolytes which will balance out your dehydration. It also helps to add magnesium, sodium, potassium, and amino acids. It also helps decrease muscle wasting, cramping, spasms, and headaches.

Sleeping eight hours a night will also help alleviate the low-energy feelings and help you not feel so drained. If you are finding it hard to sleep, try a supplement of 400 milligrams of magnesium citrate right before bedtime.

Muscle weakness

Due to the changes taking place, you may experience a change in strength that makes it harder to recover from rigorous exercise or generalized weakness. Due to this, you should withhold your rigorous exercises until you have reached a more energized state in ketosis. If you are dealing with hypoglycemia, then you should definitely take a break from exercise during the first few weeks of Keto.

There are several ways to combat this challenge. Making sure you are getting the right amount of protein is one way to ensure you are not feeling as weak. However, do not overeat protein. It may cause you to be dehydrated, have mood swings, and even kidney issues.

Increased Cravings

The advantage to eating the Keto diet is that you can cut your calorie intake without feeling ravenous. However, due to the decrease in carbs and sugars, you will find that these cravings have increased. Your dietary food patterns take time to change, and a habit takes 21 days to adjust to. It is normal to deal with some withdrawal symptoms when removing your favorite foods from your diet. Sometimes, this can be more emotional than physical so take your time and remember that you will eventually no longer have a craving for carbs and sugars. You should also remember that over time your taste buds will adjust to new flavors and preferences.

By ensuring that you are eating enough calories, you should give yourself enough time for the cravings and preferences to be sorted out. This will result in you feeling better in the long run. You should also eat more healthy fats, lean proteins, and fiber. This will help stop the cravings. If you are finding you are having cravings or stomach issues, then eating foods that are rich in probiotics should alleviate these issues.

Social Stigmas

Many people are prejudging the process of Intermittent Fasting before reading the research. As with any new diet program, people tend to naysay the benefits and deem them dangerous or not useful. So ignore the social stigma. Within a couple of years, the Intermittent Fasting craze will be upon us, and everyone will be doing it.

Healthy Eating

Although we are fasting for 16 hours, we should not just eat anything. Fasting does not make it impossible to gain weight. It is just as easy to gain weight while fasting if you are not eating a healthy diet in-between fasting. So eat your Keto diet, and be conscious of what you are putting into your body. You should always eat in moderation and follow the diet plan that you are working with. Occasionally, it doesn't hurt to treat yourself to something nice. Just don't make it a habit and derail all your progress.

Patience

Patience is the number one challenge that most people face. Everyone wants to lose weight; however, they expect it to happen overnight. This is just not possible. It takes time to lose weight. You must be patient and lose weight gradually. If you rush the weight loss, you will either harm yourself or eventually pack on those pounds. Although Intermittent Fasting will test your patience levels, you will be glad to know that you are not only losing weight but also reaping several health benefits in the process. Some of those benefits are an improved immune system, increased gut health, and autophagy. So give it time, and you will be much happier in the long run.

Crankiness

When we are hungry, we tend to get cranky. This is because our digestive system is directly connected to our nervous system. When we change our diet, the production of our hormones changes as well as our neurotransmitters. This affects our sleep and our feelings; it also affects how we behave. If you are feeling hungry or unsatisfied with your diet, you may behave irrationally. This is normal; however, you should continue to be patient with the Keto diet. It takes more than a few days to reach ketosis, and once there, you will feel better, sleep better, and behave more logically. If you are feeling sleepy, sluggish, or have a headache, and it is the cause of your nasty mood, then consider adding more magnesium to your diet. This can be done with leafy greens, avocado, and leafy vegetables. Eating at least 2 cups per day will add an extra boost to your mood. Other ways to help the mood swings is to meditate, exercise, or journal your feelings. These involve nonfood items that can improve your mood without breaking your diet.

What can you expect to experience when starting the Keto diet?

- Cramps- Leg cramps can happen early in the day or late at night. This is one challenge of the Keto diet. To stop the cramps, use potassium and drink more water. This allows the muscles to be hydrated and gives the muscles nutrients they need to stay limber. Leg cramps mean that you are needing more magnesium and potassium in your diet.

- Constipation-Constipation is the number one issue with most people who are trying to go into ketosis. The key way to alleviate this is to eat more leafy greens that are high in fiber and drink at least 1 gallon of water a day.

- Heart palpitations-This can result from stress being placed on the body. It can also be due to hypoglycemia. Drink lots of fluids and add some sodium to your diet. Make sure you are getting proper nutrients and do not overexert yourself.

- Reduced physical performance-Anytime, you start a new diet you will notice a reduction in your physical capabilities. Do not stress over this. Your body will eventually adjust to the ketosis process, and with Intermittent Fasting, it can take less time for it to adjust. This should increase your physical strength once the body adjusts.

Other side effects include:

- Increased cholesterol

- Hair loss

- Indigestion issues

- Keto rash

- Gallstones.

How to avoid the challenges that may arise

There are several challenges that can present themselves if you do not follow the Intermittent Fasting with the Keto diet properly. Oftentimes, these challenges arise due to the participant not properly following the rules. The Keto flu is one of the challenges that can happen when doing ketosis. This challenge comes when you have depleted your glucose stores, and your body is switching to ketones. One way to avoid this challenge is to use Intermittent Fasting to enhance the speed at which you reach ketosis.

A few tips on how to combat challenges that may arise on the Intermittent Fasting and Keto diet.

1. Make sure you are eating enough food during your non-fasting periods. Although Intermittent Fasting helps you eat less, you are still going to need to make sure your meals are nutritious. This will help you avoid deficiencies or metabolic issues. There are several websites that provide a calculator to calculate your ideal caloric intake and ketogenic macros needed for sustainable nutrition.

2. Make sure to measure your ketone levels while fasting. Keep an eye on how much protein and how many carbs you are eating. There are several things that can kick you out of ketosis so be careful and follow the guidelines.

So what exactly is the Keto flu?

The keto flu is the body's way of responding to the adjustment you are making by placing your body into ketosis. It comes with several symptoms that can be different for every person.

- Headaches

- Brain fog

- Severe cold symptoms

- Insomnia

- Light headedness

- Dizziness

- Constipation

- Diarrhea

- And many others

How to mitigate symptoms if they do arise

Ketosis is a metabolic change in the processing of energy in your body. When you first start the Keto diet, you should hold off on the Intermittent Fasting diet until after the first few weeks of the low carb/Keto diet. This will help you to adjust properly to the diet change. When you start the Intermittent Fasting portion of this diet, it will super boost your Ketosis, making the process more manageable, and you will be more successful with your goal. Another way to avoid challenges when on the Intermittent Fasting and Keto diet is to not to plan out everything. Listen to what your body is wanting. If it is lunch and you are not hungry, then do not eat. Wait until you are hungry. However, remember the ratio that you are aiming for with your Intermittent Fasting and keep the balance. This will help your body stay on a schedule of eating when you are supposed to be eating and fasting when you are supposed to be fasting.

Another way to avoid challenges is to not force yourself. If you are no longer hungry and your eating period is not finished yet, do not worry. You do not have to force yourself to eat. Just remember that you are not always going to get all of your caloric values every day. Some days, you are not going to be as hungry as others. Just take it slow and be mindful of your needs. You should never restrict or deprive yourself of food. However, when you first start, you are going to be struggling with the change in the eating schedule so go slow and give yourself time to adjust. Avoid snacking between meals. Snacking will derail your Intermittent Fasting and Keto diet so stay strong and do not snack a lot.

Oftentimes when we are really busy, we will forget to eat. This is okay because it gives us some fasting time. Try to keep busy in those fasting hours. This will help you to fast without being bothered by hunger. Remember the goal is to not feel hungry but to satiate yourself sufficiently during the eating state so that you no longer have a need to eat during your fasting state. Just drink lots of water and no calorie drinks while in the fasting state. You do not want to dehydrate.

Chapter 3: Challenges that You May Face with Intermittent Fasting and the Keto Diet

Another challenge that arises during the Intermittent Fasting and Keto Diet is that you may be fixed on a specific result. Do not expect this diet to fix everything. There are many factors that go into whether or not you are successful with your goals. These can range from improperly following the plan to stress levels, insufficient sleeping habits, micronutrients, macronutrients, and exercise levels. This is not a quick-fix program, and you have to be patient and willing to do what it takes to get the results you need. But never deprive yourself. If your body is craving something, you are more than likely lacking this nutrient. Eat in moderation; do not overindulge.

Brief Overview of This Chapter

- *In this chapter, we discussed challenges that you may face while being on the Intermittent Fasting and Keto diet plan.*

- *We talked about how you can avoid these challenges and how to mitigate them if they happen.*

Chapter 4:
When to Eat on the Intermittent Fasting Diet and What You Can Eat

When is it best time to eat on the Intermittent Fasting and the Keto Diet plan, and what makes this the best time?

The best times to eat during the Intermittent Fasting diet is based on when you are most active. There are several schedules that work for most people. These schedules include 12 hours, 14 hours, and 16 hours of fasting time. This allows for 10 hours and 8 hours of nutrient-based eating times.

Why certain foods are better when on the Intermittent Fasting and the Keto diet plan

When eating an Intermittent Fasting diet, there are no specific foods that are better or worse. However, we are also combining it with the Keto diet.

Under Keto, you are eating a low-carb, high-fat, and moderate-protein diet. This can be achieved by following the recommendations for the Keto diet plan.

Below we have listed foods that are acceptable and not acceptable on the Keto diet.

Here is a list of foods that are not allowed on the Keto diet.

- Grains should be avoided on the Keto diet. Grains consist of wheat, rice, corn, and cereals. Grain is also what makes bread and noodles.

- In the Keto diet, sugar is a big no-no. So is anything that is sugar-based. This includes honey, natural sweeteners, agave nectar, and maple syrup.

- Another food you should avoid on the Keto diet is fruit such as apples, bananas, and oranges due to their high-carb content.

- Potatoes and yams are full of carbs and should be avoided when on the Keto diet.

- Bulletproof coffee or buttered coffee is an absolute no-no when it comes to Intermittent Fasting. It will derail your fasting in a heartbeat due to the high caloric value.

Here is the list of allowable foods that will work on the Keto diet.

- Lean meats are a great option for the Keto diet. Meats such as fish, beef, lamb, poultry, and eggs are high in fiber and protein.

- Salads and leafy greens make for a great meal options while on the Keto diet. They provide a ton of fiber and nutrients. These can be spinach, kale, above ground vegetables, broccoli, cauliflower, and many others.

- Dairy can be a great source of fat. Creams, milk, and cheeses are good options for when you need extra protein. Add in some nuts and seeds such as macadamias, walnuts, sunflower seeds, and other nuts.

- Many people are eating avocado, and they should. It is an excellent source of protein and nutrients and makes for a great snack or meal option while on the Keto diet.

- Berries such as raspberries, blackberries, and low-glycemic fruits are another great source of nutrients.

- If you need sweeteners, then substitute your sugar for stevia, erythritol, and monk fruit for your sweeteners. They are lower glycemic and will not produce high carbs.

- Try substituting the butters and oils in your meals with olive oil and coconut oil and use some high-fat salad dressings as well as saturated fats.

Since Keto is a low-carb diet plan, there is a need for substitutes for the carbs that you are currently eating in your daily diet. Several of our favorite foods contain a lot of carbs. It is best to find a substitute that will not change the the flavor of your meals. Below is a list of carb substitutes that you can use for many recipes.

- Coconut Oil
- Cauliflower
- Kale

- Lettuce Leaves
- Portobello Mushrooms
- Spaghetti Squash
- Almond Flour Bread
- Zucchini Noodles
- Cloud Bread
- Sliced Eggplant
- Coconut Flour Bread
- Cucumber Chips
- Pork Rinds
- Kale Chips
- Cheese Chips
- Baked Carrot Sticks
- Crispy Green Beans
- Kelp Noodles
- Radish Chips
- Vegetable Noodles
- Crispy Zucchini Fries
- Stevia
- Shirataki Noodles
- Almond Milk
- Zoodles or Eggplant Noodles
- Croutons
- Fresh Crushed Tomatoes

So what can you eat with Intermittent Fasting?

The point of Intermittent Fasting is to break from eating for a specified period of time. This does not mean that you continue to eat unhealthily when you are eating. It simply means that you will eat 8 hours of the day and fast for 16 hours of the day. So how do you lose weight and maintain your health on Intermittent Fasting? The first step is to know what is healthy and how to incorporate it into your daily meals. Below we have listed several options for you. This will help you to understand more about how healthy eating works.

1. Water is a necessary part of our diets. Hydration is very important for your muscle mass and brain functions. How do you know that you are hydrated? Your urine will be a pale, yellow color. A dark, yellow color would be dehydration, and this can cause headaches, lightheadedness, and fatigue. When you add that with a limited supply of food, you have what could potentially be a recipe for disaster. If you are one of those rare people who think plain water is not flavorful, then add some slices of lemon, lime, orange, or mint leaves to the water. You can even add in some cucumber slices which add a fresher, clean taste.

2. Avocado is not a new fruit. Recently, many healthy food enthusiasts have started preaching the benefits of avocado like it is something new. Even though avocado is a high-calorie fruit, the monounsaturated fat that is found in the avocado can be extremely filling. This is a great option for those days when you need a high-calorie punch without preparing a large meal. Studies

have shown that having a half of an avocado for lunch can give you all the energy and nutrients you need to last longer during your day without the snack hunger cravings.

3. Fish is another great option for maintaining your caloric value. You should eat at least 8 oz. of fish per week. Due to its high content of protein and healthy fats, it makes an excellent meat source while on the Intermittent fasting and Keto diet. Vitamin D is a nutrient-rich vitamin and something we all could use more of. Fish contains high levels of Vitamin D, and with the limited diet on the Intermittent Fasting and Keto diet plan, you will need to get as much Vitamin D as you possibly can during your day. Fish is also great for brain functions so eat up.

4. Cruciferous vegetables like Brussel sprouts, broccoli, and cauliflower have high fiber content. When we eat on an Intermittent Fasting and Keto diet, fiber is necessary for optimum nutrients and health. So indulging in cruciferous vegetables is a great way to add more fiber to your diet. Fiber is a filler and helps you feel full for longer which is an added benefit that is necessary when fasting.

5. Beans and legumes are a great source of protein. For those who do not eat meat or meat by-products, legumes can be the protein replacement that you need. They are low-carb, making them a great option for the Keto diet, and lentils, black beans, peas, and chickpeas

have shown that they support the decrease in body weight.

6. Probiotics are microorganisms that help you with proper digestion and bowel functions. They have shown signs that they can prevent and treat some illnesses and diseases. They help with proper digestive track health and give you a support system for your immune system. They are friendly, good, and healthy bacteria. You can find them in foods such as kefir, kraut, and kombucha.

7. Berries are not only delicious but also provide vital nutrients. Strawberries have great immune-boosting vitamin C benefits; they contain more than 100% of the daily value needed in one cup. With a daily consumption of flavonoids such as blueberries and strawberries, you can decrease your BMI over a 14-year period. This helps support your weight loss efforts.

8. Eggs have 6 g of protein in one egg and can be cooked several different ways very quickly. Protein helps you stay full and build muscle so eating eggs are part of a healthy diet. When eating an egg for breakfast instead of a carb-loaded bagel, you can stay full longer and have more fuel for energy. This helps you feel less hungry throughout your day. Hard boil some eggs and divide them throughout your day as a healthy food option or snack.

9. Nuts, although high in calories, tend to be a healthy snack or garnish for many meals. It contains good fats such as polyunsaturated fat which can alter the

physiological markers that are for hunger and satiety. A 1 oz. serving of almonds contains 20% fewer calories than listed on the nutrition label. What this means is that by chewing the nuts, you are not completely breaking down the cell walls of the nut which means that you left a portion of the nut intake allowing for it to be unabsorbed during digestion.

How to design a 1-week meal plan

With the Intermittent Fasting and Keto Diet, you have several options for developing a 1-week meal plan. The important part is to follow your health needs and remember that hunger is not the goal.

How you can design an eating plan.

1. Eat from 9am-9pm, fast for 12 hours

2. Eat from 9am-7pm, fast for 14 hours

3. Eat from 12pm-8pm, fast for 16 hours

These are a few ways you can incorporate Intermittent Fasting into your Keto daily diet.

To design the meal plan, you first have to determine what and when you are going to eat. There are several cookbooks that are designed for the Keto diet. These can be used with the Intermittent Fasting and Keto diet lifestyle. Choosing what your fasting schedule will be is the first step. Then collect recipes for the meals that you will be eating so that you can arrange them in an order that works best for you. Oftentimes, we are told to eat 5-6 small meals a day. This is not the case with the Intermittent Fasting and Keto diet plan. With this plan, we are going to be eating steady meals for a specified time period.

The goal is to take in 70% high fat, 25% moderate protein, and 5% low carb. When planning your day, make sure you have these ratios in perfect proportion. These need to be eaten between the 3 meals that are designated for your non-fasting time. This will help fuel you for the fasting period and also help you reach ketosis.

Sample 1-week meal plan for Intermittent Fasting and the Keto diet

For this sample one-week meal plan, we are designing a meal plan that is for optimal health and fat reduction.

We are going to focus on the 16/8 diet. This means that we are going to only eat for 8 hours out of the day. This can be done by eating from 12pm-8pm or 10am-6pm, as well as 1-9pm. This is dependent on when you go to bed. You want to make sure you have a 4-hour window before you go to bed.

A 1-week diet plan can consist of 5 days if you are skipping the fasting on the weekend, or it can be a full 7-day Intermittent Fasting plan.

Monday:

Wake 9 am

1st meal: 1pm-2pm

Can of tuna, Greek yogurt, and berries

2nd meal: 5pm-6pm

Omelets of 2 eggs and .75 cup of egg whites, half avocado

3rd meal: 8pm-9pm

Steak and vegetables with cauliflower rice

Fasting from 9 pm until 1 pm the next day.

Tuesday:

Wake 9 am

1st meal: 1pm-2pm

Greek yogurt with berries and almonds

2nd meal: 5pm-6pm

Chicken breast, apples with cinnamon, and cottage cheese

3rd meal: 8pm-9pm

Chicken tacos with avocado salsa

Fasting from 9 pm until 1 pm the next day.

Wednesday:

Wake 9 am

1st meal: 1pm-2pm

Omelets of 2 eggs and .75 cup of egg whites, half avocado

2nd meal: 5pm-6pm

Greek yogurt with berries and avocado toast

3rd meal: 8pm-9pm

Smoked salmon with mixed green salad and vinaigrette

Fasting from 9 pm until 1 pm the next day.

Thursday:

Wake 9 am

1st meal: 1pm-2pm

Avocado salsa and eggs

2nd meal: 5pm-6pm

Jalapeno Popper soup

3rd meal: 8pm-9pm

Unstuffed pepper soup

Fasting from 9 pm until 1 pm the next day.

Friday:

Wake 9 am

1st meal: 1pm-2pm

Oatmeal with apples

2nd meal: 5pm-6pm

Chicken burritos with avocado salsa

3rd meal: 8pm-9pm

Slow cooker meat lover's pizza

Fasting from 9 pm until 1 pm the next day.

Saturday:

Wake 9 am

1st meal: 1pm-2pm

Deviled Egg salad

2nd meal: 5pm-6pm

Bruschetta Chicken

3rd meal: 8pm-9pm

Shepherd's Pie

Fasting from 9 pm until 1 pm the next day.

Sunday:

Wake 9 am

1st meal: 1pm-2pm

Chia seed pudding with berries

2nd meal: 5pm-6pm

Omelets of 2 eggs and .75 cup of egg whites, half avocado

3rd meal: 8pm-9pm

Balsamic Beef pot roast

Fasting from 9 pm until 1 pm the next day.

You can find recipes from my other book "The Complete Ketogenic Cookbook" I also have a vegan and vegetarian ketogenic cookbooks.

"Vegan Ketogenic Cookbook" – Charlotte Melhoff

"Vegetarian Ketogenic Diet Cookbook" – Charlotte Melhoff

Brief Overview of This Chapter

- *We discussed in this chapter when it is best to eat on the Intermittent Fasting diet, and what exactly is an acceptable food option. Why these foods are best and what you should avoid.*

- *Then we discussed how to design a 1-week meal plan on the Intermittent Fasting and Keto diet.*

- *Next, we gave you a sample 1-week meal plan for the Intermittent Fasting and Keto diet.*

Chapter 5:
The 16/8 diet and How You Can Use it for Your Life

The 16/8 diet is a schedule that helps you to know when you are fasting and when you are eating. In the 16/8 diet, you are fasting for 16 hours out of your awake time, and the 8 hours is the eating window when you will eat to replenish your nutrients.

This schedule can look like this:

1. Eat from 12pm-8pm, fast from 8pm-12 pm

2. You could also eat from 1pm-9pm and fast from 9pm-1pm

3. Or you could eat from 10am-6pm and fast from 6pm-10 am.

However, you design you fasting time, make sure it is during some of your active daylight time.

The part that you will need to focus on most in this diet is that you have a clear window of eating and fasting time periods. Oftentimes, people skip their breakfast and eat a larger dinner. However, studies have shown that eating later at night can increase your insulin response, allowing your fat to be stored, and increasing your waistline. They attribute this process to the circadian rhythm, which is the rhythm at which your body will know when to rise and when to rest. Because of the circadian rhythm, doctors say to eat no later than 3 hours prior to bedtime, allowing your food to digest before you lie down. Not only will this prevent you from storing the excess, but it also prevents several symptoms that you could receive if you have heartburn or GERD.

It is very crucial to your progress to eat a healthy diet during this type of fasting. That is why the Keto diet is an excellent choice for your healthy diet option during Intermittent Fasting. During your fasting time, you are not allowed to eat. However, you can drink water, tea, and coffee. The only other type of drink allowed during a fasting is bone broth. This is due to its mineral content that helps with longer fasting periods. This can help those who struggle to succeed in the longer fasting periods, 16 hours or more. It can help sustain you for the period of the fast without adding caloric value. Women who are fasting find it difficult sometimes due to the hormonal factors from a long period of no nutritional intake.

This type of fasting is suitable for those who are new to fasting or have just started fasting as well as people who are on a low-carb or Keto diet. Other people who would benefit from the 16/8 diet are people who have previous eating disorders and those that can handle fasting for more than 16 hours at a time.

Other forms of Intermittent Fasting schedules.

The 20:4 Method is a fasting protocol which is similar to the one we discussed above called the 16:8. However, the differences are that you fast for 20 hours instead of 16. You will eat the bulk of your caloric intake in a 4-hour time frame.

Because of the length of time that you have for fasting in this protocol, you should really start with another protocol of fasting before taking on this one. Most of the time, it is easier to start with a smaller fasting window. For instance, starting with just missing breakfast can help you to begin the process of acclimating to the Intermittent Fasting process.

If you choose to dive right into the 20:4 protocol, then you can expect to experience some dizziness and excessive hunger until your body reaches ketosis. This can take a bit longer especially if you are feeding those hunger pains or noshing on cravings.

There are several versions of this protocol: 17:7, 22:2, and so on. However, you break it up is up to you. Just ensure that your fasting hours are more than your eating hours.

One meal a day

The one meal a day protocol is essentially a 23:1 fasting protocol. What this means is that in one hour of the day you consume all your daily calories and macronutrients in a single meal. Due to the difficulty of overeating on this diet, you tend to see much more drastic results. Since you are only having a single meal, you cannot possible overeat or take in too many calories. Although it can be a completely natural process to eat on this schedule, you should allow yourself time to adjust to this protocol. It will take time for your body to adjust to this limited space for eating.

Recipes to help you get started on the Intermittent Fasting and the Keto Diet

Almond–Chia & Coconut Pudding

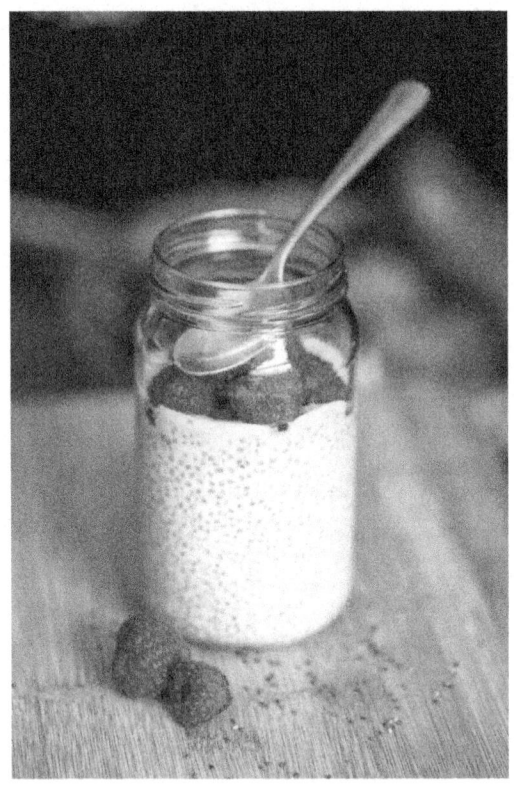

Almond Chia and coconut pudding is a great option for a snack or breakfast Keto diet meal. The pudding is low in calories which makes it a great weight loss option as well as being high in fat and protein. With only 1.5 g of net carbs, you are getting a filling breakfast with all the added health benefits.

Prep & Cook Time: 20 min.

Yields: 4 Servings

Nutrition Values:

- Calories: 130

- Fat: 12 g

- Protein: 14 g

- Net Carbs: 1.5 g

Ingredients:

- ½ c. of each:

- Chia seeds

- Chopped almonds

- ¼ c. shredded coconut

- 2 c. almond milk

Preparation Method:

1. Measure out all of your ingredients and add them to the Instant Pot while stirring. Secure your lid and select the high setting (2-5 minutes).

2. Once done cooking, press the Quick Release on the instant pot allowing the pressure to release and place the pudding into four serving glasses.

3. Top with coconut, almonds, or any other garnish.

4. Serve and enjoy!

Ketogenic Eggs

Many people eat eggs for breakfast, and this egg recipe is an exceptional example of what you can do with your eggs for the Keto diet. Their net carbs are slightly high compared to other breakfast options, but the fat content makes this meal a great option for the Keto diet.

Prep & Cook Time: 20 min.

Yields: 4 Servings

Nutrition Values:

- Fat: 14.4 g

- Protein: 7.3 g

- Net Carbs: 8.3 g

Ingredients:

- 3 tbsp. ghee

- 1 sliced jalapeno—matchstick

- 1 tbsp. chopped shallot

- 1 t. of each:

- Cumin seeds

- Ground cinnamon

- 4 eggs—beaten

- 2 coarsely chopped tomatoes

- 1 coarsely chopped green bell pepper

- ½ t. of each:

- Salt

- Turmeric

- Ground ginger

- 3 sliced garlic cloves

- ½ c. chopped cilantro

Preparation Method:

1. Add the ghee to the Instant Pot. Melt the ghee using the sauté function then add the cumin seeds, continuing to cook until aromatic.

2. Continue cooking for 3 minutes along with the shallots. Stir in the peppers, tomatoes, jalapenos, and garlic. Sauté 3 additional minutes and add the salt, ginger, and turmeric.

3. Whisk in the eggs and cook until set (30 seconds). When the eggs are at the right texture, sprinkle with the cilantro, pepper, and salt.

4. Secure the lid and cook for 13 minutes. Quick release the steam valve and serve.

Ham & Beans

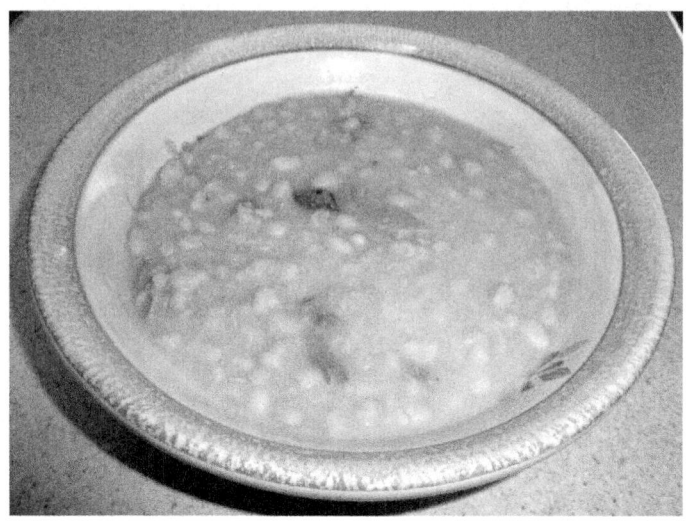

With the Keto diet, you need meals that are high in fat and low in carbs. However, after a big workout, you need to add more carbs to your diet. This meal is a great option for an after-workout carb load.

Prep & Cook Time: 1 hr. 8 min.

Yields: 6 Servings

Nutrition Values:

- Calories: 269

- Fat: 14 g

- Protein: 21 g

- Net Carbs: 13 g

Ingredients:

- 1 c. of each:
- Chopped celery
- Dried black soybeans—after soaking yields = 2 c. beans
- Chopped onion
- 1 t. of each:
- Cajun seasoning
- Dried oregano
- Liquid smoke
- Salt—maybe ½ t.
- Louisiana Hot Sauce
- 4 minced garlic cloves
- 2 smoked ham hocks
- 2 t. all-purpose seasoning
- 2 c. of each:
- Chopped ham
- Water

Preparation Method:

1. Add all of the ingredients to your Instant Pot and choose the bean/chili function (30 minutes, high-pressure). Use the natural release for 10 minutes, and then quick release the rest of the pressure in the pot.

2. Trash the bone, ensuring all the meat is off of it first. Then add the meat back into the soup. Roughly puree some of the soup with an immersion blender.

3. Enjoy piping hot garnishing with hot sauce on the side.

Cabbage Roll "Unstuffed" Soup

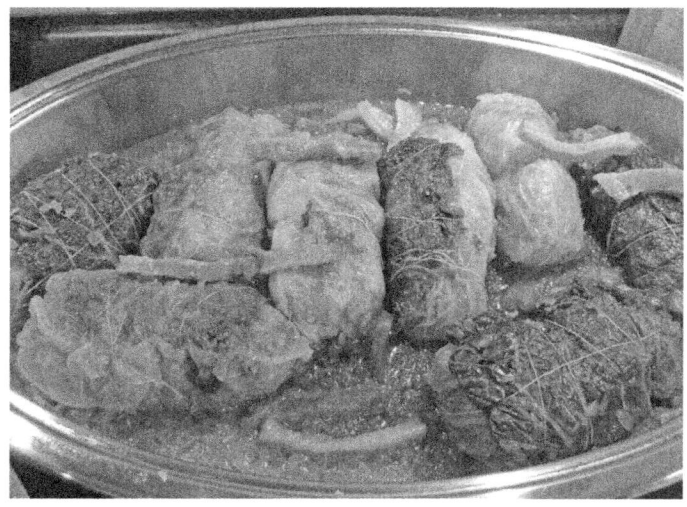

Soup is a great way to get a large number of ingredients without a lot of prep work. This meal has 217 calories which when served for lunch will help you with keeping your caloric value low during the 2nd meal of the day as well as lowering your carb intake with the 4.3 g of net carbs per serving.

Prep & Cook Time: 41 min.

Yields: 9 Servings

Nutrition Values:

- Calories: 217

- Fat: 14.8 g

- Protein: 15.6 g

- Net Carbs: 4.3 g

Ingredients:

- ½ small diced onion

- 2 minced garlic cloves

- 1 can (8oz.) tomato sauce

- 1 ½ lb. ground beef—80/20

- ¼ c. Bragg's Aminos

- 1 can diced tomatoes (14 oz.)

- 3 c. beef broth

- 3 t. Worcestershire sauce "keto" approved/another substitute

- 1 med. chopped cabbage

- ½ t. of each:

- Pepper

- Salt

- Parsley

Preparation Method:

1. Prepare using the sauté function on the Instant Pot to brown the beef, garlic, and onions. Drain this mixture and then add it back to the pot with the rest of the ingredients.

2. Program the Instant Pot to the soup function. Use the natural release valve for about 10 minutes, and quick release the rest of the steam from the soup.

3. Stir and serve.

Lunchtime Cauliflower Soufflé

You cannot go wrong with the cauliflower souffle. It has only 5 g of net carbs, which makes it an ideal option for the Keto diet as well as the low caloric value of 342 which places it right in the appropriate nutritional value for a lunch or dinner meal.

Prep & Cook Time: 32 min.

Yields: 6 Servings

Nutrition Values:

- Calories: 342

- Fat: 28 g

- Protein: 17 g

- Net Carbs: 5 g

Ingredients:

- 1 head cauliflower

- 2 eggs

- ½ c. of each:

- Sour cream/Yogurt

- Asiago cheese

- 2 tbsp. cream

- 2 oz. cream cheese

- ¼ c. chives

- 2 t. softened butter/ghee

- 1 c. mild/sharp cheddar cheese

- Optional: 6 slices crumbled cooked bacon

Preparation Method:

1. Combine the cheddar and asiago cheese along with the sour cream, cream cheese, and eggs in a food processor. Pulse until smooth and frothy.

2. Chop the cauliflower and add to the food processor (pulse 2 seconds at a time). Blend in the butter and chives. Empty into a 1 ¼-quart casserole dish.

3. Pour the water into the Instant Pot. Secure the top and cook for 12 minutes using the high-pressure setting. Use the natural release for 10 minutes, and then the quick release to release all the steam.

4. Garnish with the bacon if you choose.

5. Serve and enjoy!

Greek Meatballs With Tomato Sauce

Meatballs are everyone's favorite addition to spaghetti. With this Greek Meatball recipe, you are getting an amazing meal with only 12 g net carbs, making this an ideal low-carb meal for the Keto diet. It comes in at only 216 calories which gives you room to eat a salad or fruit along with the meatballs.

Prep & Cook Time: 40 min.

Yields: 6 Servings

Nutrition Values:

- Calories: 261

- Fat: 16 g

- Protein: 15 g

- Net Carbs: 12 g

Ingredients for the Meatballs:

- ¼ c. chopped parsley

- 1 slightly beaten egg

- 1 lb. ground beef

- 1/3 c. Arborio rice

- ½ c. finely chopped onion

- To Taste: Pepper and salt

Ingredients for the Sauce:

- 14 oz. diced tomatoes

- 1 c. water

- ½ t. of each:

- Cinnamon

- Smoked paprika

- ¼ t. ground cloves

- 1 t. dried oregano

- To Taste: More pepper & salt

Preparation Method:

1. Mix all of the meatballs fixings together, shaping into eight to ten balls. Arrange in a single layer in the pot.

2. Mix the sauce ingredients in a dish and pour over the prepared meatballs.

3. Program the Instant Pot for 15 minutes under high pressure. When done, release the pressure with the natural release option.

4. Remove the meatballs from the pot and blend the sauce until smooth with an immersion blender. Pour over the meatballs, garnish, and serve.

No-Beans Beef Chili

This chili is not only delicious but also a low carb meal making it a great addition to your Keto diet meal prep plan. Although this chili is slightly higher in calories, 326, you can still feel confident adding some leafy greens or maybe a salad with it, and it would make an amazing 3rd meal option.

Prep & Cook Time: 30 min.

Yields: 8 Servings

Nutrition Values:

- Calories: 326

- Fat: 17 g

- Protein: 23 g

- Net Carbs: 8 g

Ingredients:

- 2 cans tomato sauce—15 oz. each

- 2 lbs. beef

- 1 t. of each:

- Powdered/Dried oregano

- Tabasco sauce

- Garlic powder/ 2 minced cloves

- 5 tbsp. chili powder

- 1 can tomato paste—6 oz.

- 2 tbsp. cumin powder

- ½ c. dried onion flakes/ 1 med. onion chopped

- For Thinning: 1 c. chicken/beef broth

- 2 t. fine ground sea salt

Preparation Method:

1. Finely chop your onion. Using the sauté function on your Instant Pot so that you can brown the hamburger. Blend in the Tabasco, oregano, garlic, or onion flakes, salt, cumin, and chili powder. Mix the mixture thoroughly.

2. Empty one cup of the broth into the hamburger meat, but do not stir.

3. Pour in the tomato sauce and paste, but do not stir.

4. Close the top and use the manual high-pressure setting for 10 minutes. When done, use the natural release to release the pressure for 10 minutes; then use the quick release.

5. Stir and serve.

Slow Cooker Southwest Flank Steak

Slow cooker meals are a great way to get a delicious meal when you do not have time to stand at the stove all afternoon. This meal is a great option for the Keto diet and provides an amazing option for the 2nd or 3rd meal of your Intermittent Fasting meal plan. With only 274 calories, you are able to have a side of berries and even a salad. The carb count is low enough to fit into the guidelines for a Keto low-carb diet making this a superb addition to your Keto diet meal plan.

Prep & Cook Time: 9 hours, 10 min.

Yields: 4-6 servings

Nutritional Values:

- Calories: 274

- Fat: 10 g

- Protein: 24 g

- Net Carbs: 12 g

Ingredients:

- 1 Onion chopped

- 3 Garlic Cloves chopped, minced

- ½ tsp Salt

- 16 oz. Salsa jar chunky

- 2 tsp. Chili powder

- 1 Yellow bell pepper sliced

- ¼ tsp Pepper

- 1 Red bell pepper sliced

- Flank steak/or substitute round steak

Preparation Method:

1. Place your flank steak in your slow cooker.

2. Add some onions, peppers, and seasonings.

3. Cook on LOW for 7 to 9 hours.

4. Remove the steak and slice it into thin strips following the grain of the meat.

5. Serve the meat alone or with the veggies from slow cooker.

White Chicken Chili

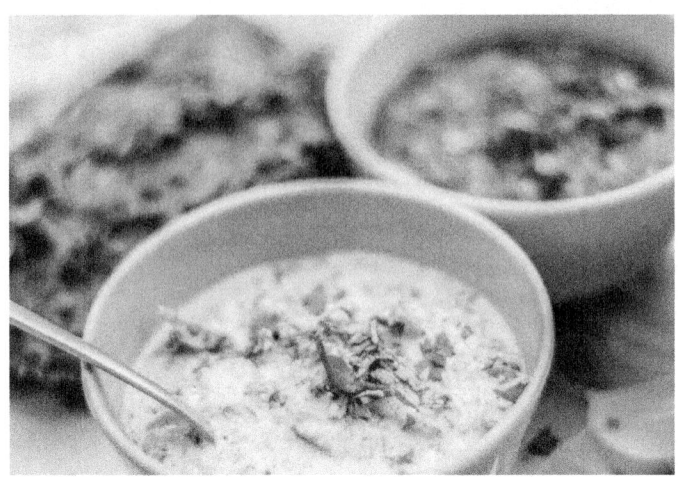

Another great chili option to use for the Keto diet. Oftentimes we look for variety in our meals. Well, this provides us a new variation to an old meal. Chili is a classic, and with this chili, you are getting no more than 6 g net carbs and only 204 calories making this an easy meal to incorporate into your Keto diet.

Prep & Cook Time: 25 min.

Yields: 4 Servings

Nutrition Values:

- Calories: 204

- Fat: 12 g

- Protein: 15 g

- Net Carbs: 6 g

Ingredients:

- 4 diced celery stalks

- 2 lb. chicken breasts—skinless—boneless

- 10 minced garlic cloves

- 2 diced onions

- 1-2 minced jalapeno peppers

- 1 t. of each:

- Cumin

- Coriander powder

- Oregano

- 1 tbsp. of each:

- Chili powder

- Salt—to taste

- 1 pkg. frozen (1 lb.) corn

- ¼ t. freshly cracked black pepper

- 4 c. chicken broth

- 1 can (15 oz.) cannellini beans—rinsed

Ingredients for Serving:

- Hot Sauce

- Cilantro

Preparation Method:

1. Mix everything into the Instant Pot (except the beans and corn).

2. Secure the lid and set the instant pot on high pressure for 15 minutes.

3. Use the quick release to release the pressure and shred the chicken in the pot, adding the corn and cannellini beans. Sauté for 5 minutes until heated.

4. Serve.

Chipotle Shredded Beef

Chipotle is a favorite of anyone who loves southwestern food, and this one does not disappoint. The calories are a little bit higher making it a great 2nd or 3rd meal option for the day. With the carb count at 2.2 g net carbs, you definitely cannot go wrong with this meal.

Prep & Cook Time: 1 hr. 35 min.

Yields: 16 Servings

Nutrition Values:

- Calories: 334

- Fat: 25.6 g

- Protein: 22.6 g

- Net Carbs: 2.2 g

Ingredients:

- 3 lb. beef chuck roast

- 2 tbsp. olive oil

- 2 t. salt

- 1 t. black pepper

- 1 chipotle in adobo—seeds removed or not—chopped

- 1 tbsp. adobo sauce—from chipotle with adobe can

- 2 t. dried of each:

- Cumin

- Oregano

- ½ t. chili powder

- 1 peeled – quartered onion

- 1 c. fresh cilantro—roughly chopped

- 1 c. water

- 1 seeded green bell pepper—large chunks

Preparation Method:

1. Sprinkle the roast with the pepper and salt for seasoning. Choose the Instant Pot's sauté function and pour in some oil. Arrange the roast in the pot and sauté 3-4 minutes on each side.

2. Spread with the adobo sauce and chipotle pepper. Sprinkle with the chili powder, cumin, and oregano. Toss the cilantro on top. Add the peppers and onions. Pour the water into the pot.

3. Cook for 60 minutes using the high-pressure setting. Use the natural release valve to release the pressure. Then remove the meat from the pot. Shred with two forks and discard the veggies.

4. Add the beef back into the juices. Keep warm until ready to serve.

Shepherd's Pie

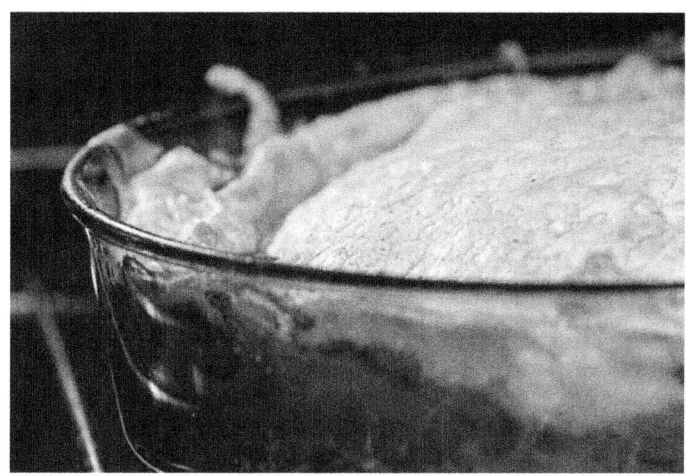

Shepherd's pie is a favorite of many who have traveled to Europe. It has a classic, full flavor that is filling and nutritious. With only 4.1 g of net carbs, this meal is a low-carb option, and only 303 calories make it a healthy option for any 2nd or 3rd meal in your Keto meal plan.

Prep & Cook Time: 45 min.

Yields: 12 Servings

Nutrition Values:

- Calories: 303

- Fat: 21.2 g

- Protein: 21.5 g

- Net Carbs: 4.1 g

Ingredients:

- 1 c. water
- 1 c. mozzarella
- 4 tbsp. butter
- 1 head cauliflower
- 4 oz. cream cheese
- 1 tbsp. garlic powder
- 2 lb. ground beef
- 1 egg
- Pepper & Salt to taste
- 2 c. of each:
- Frozen carrots
- Frozen peas
- 1 c. beef broth
- 8 oz. sliced mushrooms

Preparation Method:

1. Pour the water into the Instant Pot and layer the cauliflower on top without the stems and leaves. Close the lid and set the temperature for 5 minutes using high pressure.

2. Use the quick release valve. Next, add the cauliflower to a blender. Then add the butter, cream cheese, mozzarella, salt, pepper, and egg. Blend until smooth.

3. Drain the water from the Instant Pot. Toss in the beef, peas, carrots, garlic powder, and broth with a bit more pepper and salt to your liking.

4. Blend in the cauliflower mixture and cook for 10 minutes on high (manual function).

5. Serve and enjoy!

3- Ingredient Slow Cooker Apricot Salmon

Salmon is a great source of Omega-3s and is high in protein and fat. This recipe is only 190 calories and has 14 g net carbs. The carbs are slightly higher so this would be great after a workout.

Prep & Cook Time: 1 hour 35 min.

Yields: 2 servings

Nutrition Values:

- Calories: 190

- Protein: 24g

- Fat: 4.2g

- Net Carbs: 14g

Ingredients:

- 8 oz. Salmon, frozen wild (do NOT thaw)

- 3 tbsp Apricot fruit spread

- 4 tbsp Salsa verde

Preparation Method:

1. Grease the inside of the slow cooker with some oil to prevent sticking.

2. Place the frozen salmon in the cooker, making sure the skin side is down to ensure an evenly cooked fish.

3. Mix together your fruit spread with your salsa.

4. Spread your salsa mixture over the salmon.

5. On LOW, cook for 1-1.5 hours.

Honey Mustard Chicken, Bacon, & Avocado Salad

With the words chicken, bacon, and avocado in the recipe, you can't go wrong. This recipe is a great Keto option for adding high fat and protein. The calories of 410 make it a great 3rd meal option. Although the carbs are slightly high at 34 g net carbs, it is still a great way to get lots of nutrients.

Prep & Cook Time: 40 min.

Yields: 4 servings

Nutritional Values:

- Calories: 410

- Protein: 25g

- Fat: 20g

- Net Carbs: 34g

Ingredients:

- 4 Boneless chicken thighs or chicken breasts/thighs

- Dressing / Marinade:

- 1/3 cup Honey

- 3 tbsp Whole grain mustard

- 2 tbsp Dijon mustard

- 2 tbsp Olive oil

- 1-2 tbsp Apple cider vinegar

- 1 tbsp Garlic minced

- Salt -to taste

- For Salad:

- ¼ cup Bacon diced

- 4 cups Romaine lettuce leaves washed

- 1 cup Grapes or cherry tomatoes sliced

- 1 large Avocado pitted and sliced

- ½ cup Corn kernels

- ½ cup Red onion sliced

Preparation Method:

1. Whisk the dressing ingredients together.

2. 30 minutes prior to cooking, pour half of the dressing into a dish to marinate the chicken.

3. Heat a tsp. of oil in a pan.

4. Sear each side of the chicken until it is cooked thoroughly.

5. Once all the chicken is cooked, set it aside to rest.

6. Use a paper towel to wipe the pan out then add another tsp. of oil.

7. Cook the bacon until crispy.

8. Cut the chicken into small strips and prepare a salad with lettuce, avocado slices, tomatoes, onion strips, corn, and chicken strips.

5-Spice Slow Cooker Pork Ribs

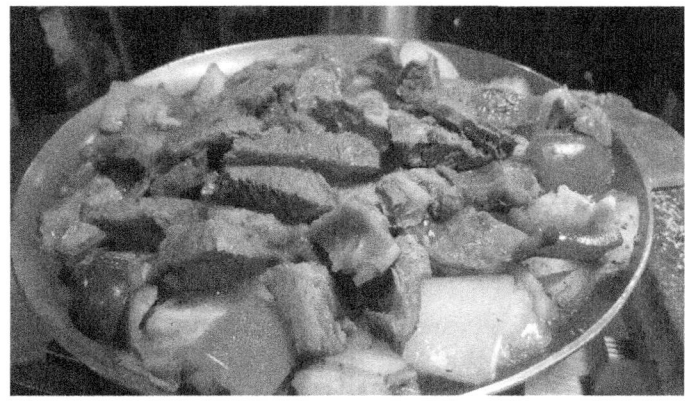

Spicy food is loved by most people so we included this spicy pork ribs meal for you to have variety with your foods. This meal is a great option because it only has 355 calories and 20 g net carbs. This also makes a great after-workout meal for boosting those fats and calories.

Prep & Cook Time: 6 hours and 2 min.

Yields: 4 servings

Nutritional Values:

- Calories: 355

- Protein: 29 g

- Fat: 17 g

- Net Carbs: 20 g

Ingredients:

- ¾ tsp Garlic powder granulated
- 2 tbsp Coconut aminos
- 2 tbsp Rice vinegar
- 1 Jalapeño fresh, cut into rings
- 2 tbsp Chinese five-spice powder
- Salt and Pepper to taste/ground black pepper
- 3-4 lbs. Baby Back or St. Louis pork ribs

Preparation Method:

1. Cut the ribs into chunks that can stand in the cooker.

2. Season the ribs with salt and pepper.

3. Mix the five-spices and garlic powder in a small bowl then rub the spices evenly onto the ribs.

4. Put the jalapeño rings in the cooker.

5. Add the tomato paste, vinegar, and aminos.

6. Mix until everything is completely blended.

7. Add the ribs to the slow cooker. Stand them up so they are not lying in the liquid.

8. On HIGH, cook for 6 hours or 8 to 10 hours on LOW.

9. Remove the ribs when they are tender and falling apart.

10. Pour the remaining liquid from the crockpot into a safe container and put in the refrigerator until the fat and juices separate.

11. Once separated, using a slotted spoon, remove the fat and bring the remaining liquid to a boil in a pot.

12. Let boil for a few minutes then drizzle over the top of the ribs.

Deviled Egg Salad

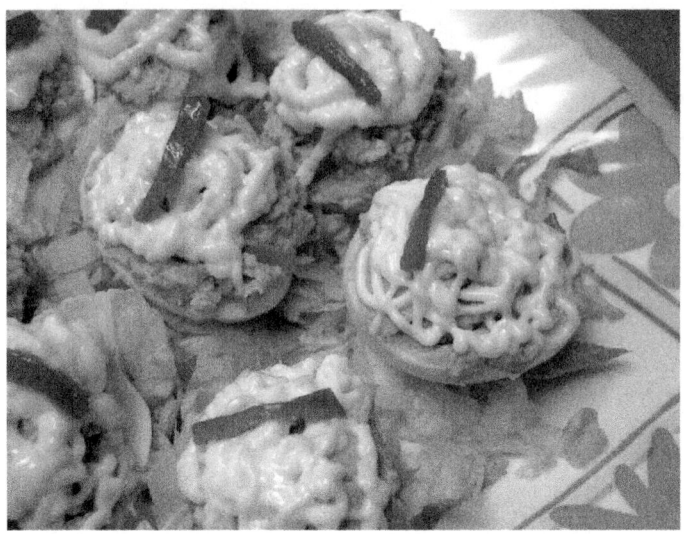

Eggs are a great breakfast option. Most people who are doing the Intermittent Fasting with the Keto diet skip breakfast. However, that doesn't mean that you have to miss out on those great meals. Eggs are great for adding fat and protein to a meal and are low in carbs.

Prep & Cook Time: 30 min.

Yields: 5 Servings

Nutrition Values:

- Calories: 313

- Fat: 26.4 g

- Protein: 16.4 g

- Net Carbs: 1.3 g

Ingredients:

- 2 tbsp. mayo

- 5 raw bacon strips

- 10 large eggs

- ¼ t. smoked paprika

- Pepper & Salt to taste

- 1 t. Dijon mustard

- 1 stalk green onion

- Also Needed: 6-7-inch cake pan

Preparation Method:

1. Grease all sides of the pan that will sit inside of the pot on the rack. Pour one cup of cold water in the bottom of the Instant Pot and add the steam rack.

2. Crack the eggs into the pan (try not to break the yolks).

3. Place the pan on the rack. Secure the lid and set the timer for 6 minutes (high-pressure). Use the natural release valve to release the pressure and remove the pan.

4. Dab away any moisture. Flip the pan on a cutting board allowing it to release from the pan. Chop the egg loaf and add to a mixing dish.

5. Clean the Instant Pot bowl and sauté the ingredients (medium heat). Cook the bacon until crispy.

6. Add mayo, mustard, pepper, paprika, and salt to the chopped eggs. Toss the mix and then garnish with green onion.

7. Serve the way you like it!

Mutton Curry

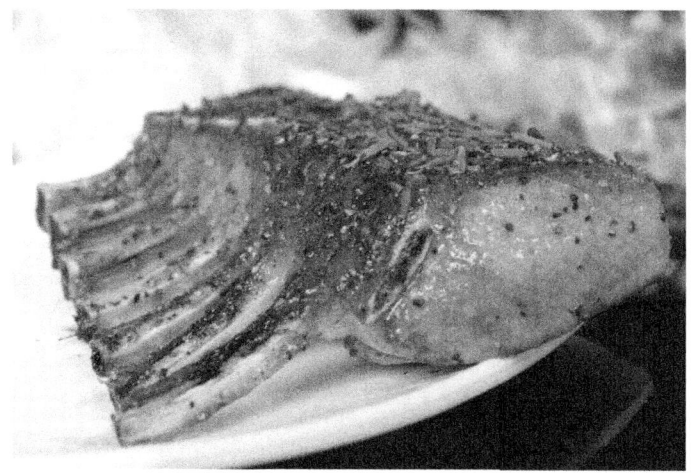

Mutton is a classic meal, and many people have been serving it for years. This recipe is a great option for a healthy, hearty meal. With only 253 calories, you can definitely add a salad to this dinner along with some side vegetables and fruit. The carb value is low, allowing you to eat this often.

Prep & Cook Time: 40 min.

Yields: 4 Servings

Nutrition Values:

- Calories: 253

- Fat: 13.5 g

- Protein: 24.65 g

- Net Carbs: 6.34 g

Ingredients:

- 1 large (11 oz.) finely chopped onion
- 3 tbsp. oil/ghee
- 1 lb. mutton bone-in (1-2-inch bits)
- Optional: 1 green chili
- ½ tbsp. minced of each:
- Garlic
- Ginger
- 1 med. chopped tomato
- 1 tbsp. lemon juice
- Garnish: Cilantro

Spices:

- 2 t. coriander
- 1 t. of each:
- Garam masala
- Cayenne/red chili powder
- Salt
- ¼ t. turmeric

Whole Spices:

- 6 of each:

- Black peppercorns

- Cloves

- 1 (1-inch) cinnamon stick

- ½ t. cumin seeds

- 1 bay leaf

- 2 black cardamom

Preparation Method:

1. Use the sauté function on the Instant Pot and pour in your oil. Throw in the whole spices and sauté them for 30 seconds. Next add in the onions, green chilies, and garlic. Sauté while stirring for 4 minutes.

2. Blend in your spices and chopped tomatoes, continue stirring for 2 minutes.

3. Stir in the mutton and mix it well, sautéing for another 2 minutes.

4. Close the lid and change the setting to the meat function for 20 minutes.

5. Use the natural release valve to release the pressure and add the lemon juice. Garnish with the mutton curry and cilantro. Enjoy!

French Garlic Chicken

This meal is a delicious variation on traditional chicken. With 429 calories, it is healthy and hearty. The 4 g of net carbs makes it an amazing option for the Keto diet, can be combined with vegetables and a side salad, and make a hearty dinner that will fill you up for a long time.

Prep & Cook Time: 30 min.

Yields: 4 Servings

Nutrition Values:

- Calories: 429

- Fat: 37 g

- Protein: 19 g

- Net Carbs: 4 g

Ingredients for the Marinade:

- 2 t. Herbes de Provence

- 2 tbsp. olive oil

- 1 tbsp. of each:

- Prepared Dijon mustard

- Minced garlic

- Cider vinegar

- 1 t. of each:

- Salt

- Pepper

- 1 lb. chicken thighs—no bones or skin

Other Ingredients:

- 2 tbsp. butter

- 8 chopped garlic cloves

- ¼ c. of each:

- Water

- Cream

Preparation Method:

1. Prepare your marinade: Add all of the ingredients using a whisk. Add the chicken and marinate for 30 minutes at room temperature. (Place in the fridge if it will take longer.)

2. Choose the sauté button and melt the butter. Sauté the garlic for 2-3 minutes.

3. Toss your chicken in the butter. Reserve the marinade. Lightly brown the chicken on each side. Pour the water and marinade into the pot and secure the lid. Cook for 10 minutes and check the temperature. (Internal temperature must be 165° F.)

4. Transfer the chicken to a plate and then add the cream to the Instant Pot, mixing it well.

5. Serve with the sauce and enjoy.

Spicy Pork—Korean Style

If you love Korean food, then this spicy pork will satiate that need. It has 189 calories per serving and only 9 g net carbs. This is an easy meal to add to any other side dishes of a Korean buffet.

Prep & Cook Time: 40 min.

Yields: 4 Servings

Nutrition Values:

- Calories: 189

- Fat: 10 g

- Protein: 15 g

- Net Carbs: 9 g

Ingredients:

- 1 thinly sliced onion

- 1 lb. pork shoulder

- 1 tbsp. of each:

- Minced garlic

- Sesame oil

- Rice wine

- Minced ginger

- Soy sauce

- 2 tbsp. Gochugaru Chili flakes

- 2 Splenda packs

- ¼ c. water

- 1 t. Cayenne

Ingredients for Finishing:

- 1 thinly sliced onion

- ¼ c. sliced green onion

- 1 tbsp. sesame seeds

Preparation Method:

1. Cut the pork into ¼- to ½-inch slices, and add the rest of the marinade ingredients into a container along with the pork. Let this rest from 1 hour to 24 hours in the fridge. When ready to cook, use the high-pressure setting for 20 minutes. Use the natural release valve to release the pressure when it is done.

2. Use a cast-iron skillet to cook the thinly sliced onion and pork cubes. Once the pan is hot, just empty in the sauce, and mix with the pork.

3. When the sauce has cooled down, the onions will be soft. Toss the green onions and sesame seeds for garnish.

4. Serve and enjoy!

Slow Cooker Crack Chicken

Crack chicken is an easy recipe to follow and has only 410 calories per serving. This meal is loaded with fat and protein and low in carbs with only 4 g. You could eat this chicken for several days on the Keto diet.

Cook & Prep Time: 8 hours and 15 min.

Yields: 8 servings

Nutritional Value:

- Calories: 410

- Protein: 28 g

- Fat: 32 g

- Net Carbs: 4 g

Ingredients:

- 8 Bacon crumbled

- 2 -8 oz. Cream cheese blocks

- 2 Ranch dressing seasoning packets

- Chicken breasts frozen

Preparation Method:

1. Lay the chicken into the slow cooker.

2. Shake the ranch dressing mix over the top of the chicken.

3. Place both blocks of cream cheese on top of the chicken.

4. On LOW, cook the chicken for 8 hours.

5. Just before serving, shred the chicken with two forks, and mix the cream cheese in with everything in the slow cooker.

6. Microwave or fry the bacon in a pan.

7. Crumble the bacon and stir it into the chicken.

8. Serve and enjoy!

Seasoned Citrus Tilapia

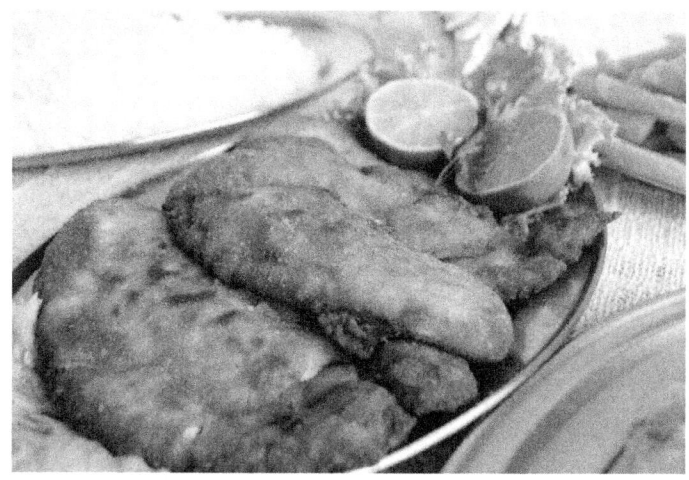

Tilapia is a light and airy fish that is low in carbs and high in protein. The calories in this meal are only 130, making this an easy recipe to mix with a side of vegetables and some fruit. This fish is perfect for the Keto diet.

Cook & Prep Time: 2 hours, 5 min.

Yields: 4 servings

Nutritional Values:

- Calories: 130

- Protein: 23 g

- Fat: 3 g

- Net Carbs: 5 g

Ingredients:

- Salt and pepper -to taste

- 1 -10 oz. Mandarin oranges drained

- 2 tbsp. Garlic butter chopped into small pieces

- 4 Tilapia fillets

- Aluminum foil

Preparation Method:

1. Set out a large piece of foil.

2. Place the fish fillets next to each other on the foil.

3. Place scoops of garlic butter evenly over the top of the fillets.

4. Place about ¼ c of oranges on each fillet.

5. Sprinkle each fillet with pepper and salt.

6. Fold the foil to seal everything in like an envelope.

7. Place the fish in the slow cooker and cook on HIGH for 2 hours.

8. Remove the fish and serve hot.

Egg Cups & Cheese

As we stated before, eggs are a staple in everyone's diet unless you do not eat animal by-products. The calories in this meal are only 115 making this an easy meal to add to some avocado or berries. With 2 net carbs, it is a great keto option.

Prep & Cook Time: 15 min.

Yields: 4 Servings

Nutrition Values:

- Calories: 115

- Fat: 9 g

- Protein: 9 g

- Net Carbs: 2 g

Ingredients:

- 1 c. diced veggies—for example, tomatoes, mushrooms, etc.

- 4 eggs

- ½ c. sharp, shredded cheddar cheese

- 2 tbsp. cilantro—chopped

- ¼ c. Half & Half

- Pepper & Salt to taste

Ingredients for the Topping:

- ½ c. shredded cheese of your choice

Also Needed:

- 2 c. water

- 4 wide-mouthed jars

Preparation Method:

1. Whisk the Half & Half, veggies, eggs, salt, pepper, cilantro, and cheese.

2. Combine the mixture into each of the jars. Securing the lids (not too tight) to keep water from getting into the egg mix.

3. Arrange the wire rack in the Instant Pot and add water. Arrange the jars on the wire rack and set the timer for 5 minutes (high pressure). When done, use the quick release valve to release the pressure, and top with the rest of the cheese (½ cup).

4. Broil if you like for 2-3 minutes until the cheese is browned to your liking.

Sausage Cheese Ring

Sausage and cheese ring is a great way to start your day. The calories are a bit higher than the 400 calories that we would allot for the 1st meal of the day. However, we can adjust our 2nd meal calories to make it a well-rounded meal plan. This meal only has 3.6 g net carbs which makes it an ideal Keto diet meal option.

Prep & Cook Time: 50 min.

Yields: 4-6 Servings

Nutrition Values:

- Calories: 470

- Fat: 35.9 g

- Protein: 28.5 g

- Net Carbs: 3.6 g

Ingredients:

- 1 lb. breakfast sausage

- 2 ½ tbsp. coconut oil

- 2 red bell peppers—½-inch cut

- 4 ½ tbsp. shredded parmesan cheese

- 4 large eggs

- Ground pepper and salt—to taste

Preparation Method:

1. Warm up the coconut oil in the Instant Pot. Then add in the pepper pieces.

2. Slice the sausages into ringlets and sauté for 2-5 minutes. Set them aside.

3. Add 4 pepper ringlets into the pot. Then add the egg to a dish and slide it into the center of the pepper ring. Season with pepper and salt. Do this with each one. Place the sausages on top (10-15 minutes).

4. Remove the rings and serve with the cheese topping.

Paprika Boiled Eggs

Paprika adds a kick to this egg recipe, making it a good spicy alternative for a lunch or 3rd mealtime option. With the calories at only 72 g and the net carbs at .4 g, you can definitely eat more than one of these or add it to some avocado and vegetables. making this a great lunch option.

Prep & Cook Time: 30 min.

Yields: 3 Servings

Nutrition Values:

- Calories: 72

- Fat: 5 g

- Protein: 6.3 g

- Net Carbs: 0.4 g

Ingredients:

- 6-8 eggs (from the fridge is okay)

- 1 c. cold water

- Paprika

Preparation Method:

1. Add the water to the Instant Pot stainless bowl and insert the steamer basket. Gently place the eggs into the basket and close the lid.

2. Set the timer for 5-10 minutes. Use the quick release valve and release the pressure then remove the eggs. When done, place in an ice-cold bath to cool. Once cooled, peel them.

3. Arrange the eggs on a serving platter and sprinkle with the paprika.

Slow Cooker Pot Roast

A pot roast is always a staple in any family menu. This pot roast is keto friendly with only 150 calories per serving and 0 g net carbs; you can eat as much as you like.

Cook & Prep Time: 9 hours and 5 min.

Yields: 4 servings

Nutritional Values:

- Calories: 150

- Protein: 24 g

- Fat: 5 g

- Net Carbs: 0 g

Ingredients:

- 3-5 lb. Chuck roast

- 2 stalks Celery cut into pieces

- White onion small, quartered

- 3 tbsp. Worcestershire sauce

- ½ tsp Garlic minced

- ¼ tsp Black pepper

- ½ tsp Parsley dried

- 4 tbsp. Butter cut into pieces

Preparation Method:

1. Place vegetables (celery and onion) in the slow cooker.

2. On top of the vegetables, place your roast.

3. Combine 3 tbsp of Worcestershire sauce, pepper, garlic, and parsley in a bowl. Stir to blend it together.

4. Pour the mixture over the roast.

5. Place butter on top.

6. On LOW, cook for 8 to 9 hours.

7. Remove roast and veggies from the slow cooker and place on a platter for serving.

8. Serve and enjoy!

Seafood Stew

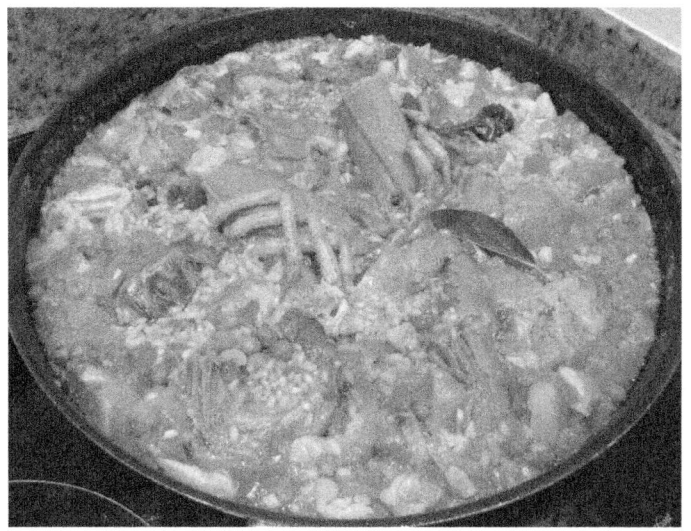

Seafood is a great meal option and really rounds out your weekly meal plans for the Keto diet. It provides you with only 8 g net carbs and 310 calories, making it hearty and filling.

Cook & Prep Time: 7 hours, 10 min.

Yields: 8 servings

Nutritional Value:

- Calories: 310

- Protein: 42 g

- Fat: 4 g

- Net Carbs: 8 g

Ingredients:

- ¼ tsp. Red pepper flakes

- 1 -28 oz. can Crushed tomatoes

- 4 cups Vegetable broth

- ½ cups White wine

- 2-3 Garlic cloves minced

- ½ lbs. Zucchini cut into bite-sized pieces

- 1 pinch Cayenne pepper

- ½ lbs. Summer squash cut into bite-sized pieces

- ½ Onion medium, diced

- 1 tsp. Dried thyme

- 2 lbs. Seafood

- 1 tsp. Dried basil

- 1 tsp. Dried cilantro

- ½ tsp. of each of these:

- Celery salt

- Salt

- Pepper

Preparation Method:

1. Add all the ingredients to the slow cooker except for the seafood.

2. On HIGH, cook for 2 to 3 hours or LOW for 4-6 hours.

3. On HIGH, add the seafood and cook for another 30-60 minutes.

Jalapeno Popper Soup

This soup is a wonderful option for that midday meal. Whether you eat it for your 1st, 2nd, or 3rd meal, you cannot go wrong with this soup. There are 571 calories in this soup. Even though it is hearty, make sure you adjust your caloric intake for the rest of the day so that you do not overeat. At 2.1 g of net carbs, you are doing good when adding this soup to your meal plan.

Prep & Cook Time: 52 min.

Yields: 8 Servings

Nutrition Values:

- Calories: 571

- Fat: 40.1 g

- Protein: 41.2 g

- Net Carbs: 2.1 g

Ingredients:

- ½ lb. Bacon—cooked and crumbled

- 1 ½ lb. Chicken breasts (boneless skinless)

- 2 Minced garlic cloves

- ½ c. Heavy whipping cream

- 3 tbsp. Butter

- ½ Chopped onion

- ½ Chopped green pepper

- 3 c. Chicken broth

- 2 Jalapenos—seeded and chopped

- 6 oz. Cream cheese

- ½ t. Pepper

- 1 t. of each:

- Cumin

- Salt

- ½ t. Xanthan gum

- ¼ t. Paprika

- ¾ c. of each cheese:

- Monterey Jack

- Cheddar

Preparation Method:

1. Prepare your Instant Pot using the sauté function. Then add the onions, butter, green peppers, jalapenos, and the seasoning. Sauté until translucent. Stir in the previously cubed chicken, broth, and cream cheese.

2. Set the timer for 15 minutes—manual. Allow for 5 minutes for the natural release valve to release the steam. Quick release after that time until fully released.

3. Next, choose the sauté function again and remove the chicken from the bone using two forks. Add the chicken, whipping cream, both kinds of cheese, and the cooked bacon. Sprinkle in the xanthan gum; this will thicken the soup.

4. Simmer for a few minutes and serve with some grated cheese, jalapenos, or bacon on the top.

Chicken Stew

Chicken stew is a great way to get lots of nutrients in a small bowl. This meal has only 290 calories and 3 g of net carbs. However, there is nothing light about this meal. It is filling and flavorful.

Prep & Cook Time: 50 min.

Yields: 8 Servings

Nutrition Values:

- Calories: 290

- Fat: 37 g

- Protein: 27 g

- Net Carbs: 3 g

Ingredients:

- 2 lb. Cut-up chicken

- 3 Diced carrots

- 2 Diced celery stalks

- 2 Bay leaves

- 8-12 c. Liquid—broth or water

- 1 Diced onion

- Fresh herbs to taste—sage, rosemary, or basil

Preparation Method:

1. Use the sauté function on your Instant Pot to prepare the celery, onions, and carrots until they are aromatic.

2. Toss in the rest of the ingredients and secure the lid.

3. Cook for 35 minutes using the high-pressure setting.

4. Use the natural release valve for releasing the pressure and serve.

Chicken Mushroom Soup

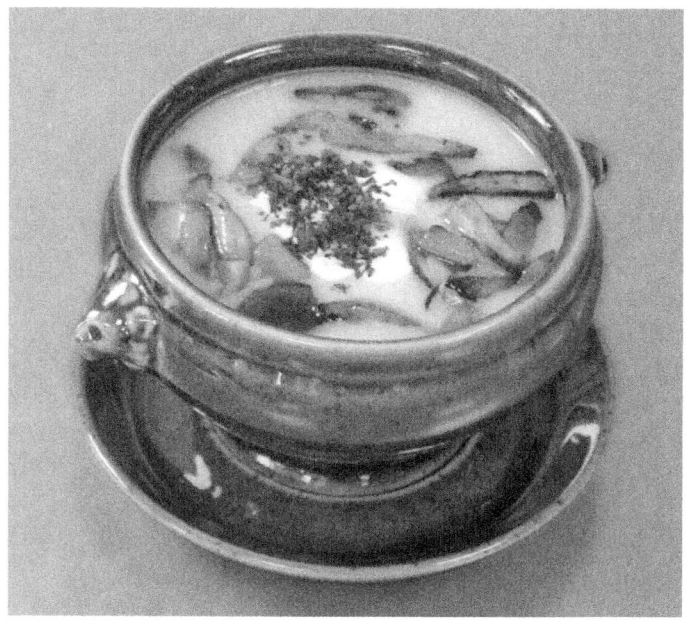

If you like mushrooms, then you will love this soup. It is packed full of nutrients and flavor. It has only 289 calories and about 9 g net carbs, making this an optimal recipe for the Keto diet.

Prep & Cook Time: 31 min.

Yields: 4 Servings

Nutrition Values:

- Calories: 289

- Fat: 15 g

- Protein: 30 g

- Net Carbs: 9 g

Ingredients:

- 1 Chopped yellow squash

- 3 Minced garlic cloves

- 1 Thinly sliced onion

- 2 ½ c. Chicken stock

- 1 t. Poultry/Italian Seasoning

- 2 c. Mushrooms—chopped

- 1 lb. Chicken breasts—remove bones and skin

- Pepper & Salt

- Optional: ½ c. Heavy whipping cream

Preparation Method:

1. Toss everything into your Instant Pot and cook for 15 minutes under high pressure. Use the natural release for 10 minutes, allowing the pressure to release, then use the quick release to finish it.

2. Remove the chicken and roughly puree the veggies with an immersion blender.

3. Shred the chicken and add it back to the cooker.

4. Add the cream, stir, and serve.

Lemon Rotisserie Chicken

Rotisserie chicken is a flavorful and fun dish to serve for your family. This one only has 284 calories and 2.9 g net carbs, making this an excellent option for the Keto diet.

Prep & Cook Time: 40 min.

Yields: 6 Servings

Nutrition Values:

- Calories: 284

- Fat: 18.8 g

- Protein: 25.7 g

- Net Carbs: 2.9 g

Ingredients:

- 4 Lemon wedges—1 lemon

- 2.5 lb. Whole chicken

- 2 tbsp. Olive oil

- 1 ½ t. Salt

- 1 t. of each:

- Garlic powder

- Paprika

- 1 c. Chicken broth

- ½ t. Ground black pepper

Preparation Method:

1. Wash the chicken and pat it dry with a paper towel. Insert lemon wedges into the cavity of the bird.

2. Choose the sauté function on the Instant Pot.

3. Combine the garlic powder, pepper, salt, oil, and paprika in a dish. Rub the top of the chicken (breast side down) using ½ of the spice mixture.

4. Sauté the chicken for 3 to 4 minutes.

5. Rub the rest on the other half and flip, cooking 1 more minute.

6. Transfer the chicken to a container and add the wire rack to the instant pot. Put the chicken on the rack (breast side down), and cover with the broth.

7. Secure the lid and set the timer for 20 minutes. Using the natural release valve, release the pressure at the end of the cooking cycle.

8. Serve and enjoy!

Beef Tips Stroganoff

Beef stroganoff has never been better. When you take a classic and make it better, you can't help but share it with others. This recipe is healthy with only 321 calories and perfect for the Keto diet since it only contains 7 g net carbs.

Prep & Cook Time: 38 min.

Yields: 4 Servings

Nutrition Values:

- Calories: 321

- Fat: 16 g

- Protein: 33 g

- Net Carbs: 7 g

Ingredients:

- 1 tbsp. of each:

- Worcestershire sauce

- Oil

- Garlic

- ½ c. Diced onions

- 1 t. Salt

- ½ t. Pepper to taste

- 1 ½ c. Chopped mushrooms

- 1 lb. Beef/pork stew meat

- ¾ c. water

Ingredients to Finish:

- 1/3 c. Sour cream

- ¼ t. Arrowroot starch/cornstarch/xanthan gum

Preparation Method:

1. Heat your Instant Pot using the sauté function. Heat the oil and toss in the garlic and onions. Stir a minute, then add the rest of the ingredients except for the sour cream.

2. Secure the lid and set on high pressure for 20 minutes. Allow the natural release to release the pressure.

3. Change to the sauté function and stir in the sour cream. Sprinkle in the xanthan gum slowly, stirring as it thickens.

4. Serve and enjoy with some low-carb noodles or cauliflower rice but add the carbs.

Carnitas

Carnitas are a popular meal option for those who love to eat. This recipe is a great keto option since it is only 1 g carbs and has 160 calories. This healthy meal can be enjoyed anytime within your non-fasting hours, making this a versatile meal option.

Prep & Cook Time: 1 hr. 16 min.

Yields: 11 Servings

Nutrition Values:

- Calories: 160

- Fat: 7 g

- Protein: 20 g

- Net Carbs: 1 g

Ingredients:

- 2 ½ lb. Shoulder blade roast—trimmed and boneless

- ½ t. Sazon GOYA

- 2 t. Kosher salt

- ½ t. Garlic powder

- ¼ t. Dry oregano

- 1 ½ t. Cumin

- Black pepper—to your liking

- 6 Minced garlic cloves

- 2-3 Chipotle peppers in adobo sauce—to taste

- ¼ t. Dry adobo seasoning—for example, Goya

- ¾ c. Reduced-sodium chicken broth/homemade

- 2 Bay leaves

Preparation Method:

1. Season the roast with pepper and salt. Sear it for about 5 minutes in a skillet on each side.

2. Let it cool and insert your garlic slivers into the roast by using a blade to cut a space out of the roast. (approximately 1-inch deep). Season with the oregano, garlic powder, cumin, sazon, and adobo.

3. Lay the chicken in the Instant Pot, and add the broth along with the chipotle peppers and bay leaves. Stir and secure the lid. Prepare using high pressure for 50 minutes (meat button).

4. Allow the natural release valve to release the pressure and shred the pork. Combine with the juices and discard the bay leaves.

5. Add a bit more cumin and adobo if needed.

6. Stir well and serve.

Brief Overview of this chapter

- *In this chapter, we discussed the 16/8 diet and several variations of the Intermittent Fasting and Keto diet. We talked about the benefits and how to make a schedule for fasting that works.*

- *Then we discussed recipes to get you started on the Intermittent Fasting and Keto diet and explained why each meal is a great choice for your meal plan.*

Chapter 6:
How to fit this diet into your needs

How can exercise help you?

Exercise is good for everyone, and when using the Intermittent Fasting and keto diet plan, you can work exercise into your fasting plan fairly easily. Many people have found that they get more benefits from exercise they do while fasting. There is scientific proof that states that you get the maximum fat-burning benefits especially after using cardio. However, this will vary per person. The participants who are doing the 16:8 and 20:4 have seen greater benefits. Those who are participating in the 24 hour or extended fasting should not exercise on their fasting days. This can cause a large spread of adrenal fatigue and do more harm than good.

How can you incorporate Intermittent Fasting into your work day along with the Keto diet?

Intermittent Fasting is not always easy. However, if you are anything like most people, you find yourself not eating when you are busy. This is how you are going to be able to incorporate Intermittent Fasting and the Keto diet into your workday. When you get up first thing in the morning, at this time, you should be fasting. You have already prepared a meal the night before to bring with you to work for both your first meal and your second meal. Instead of drinking coffee with sugar and cream, drink black coffee or water for your morning commute. You get to work at 7 or 8 am, and you go straight to working on whatever your tasks are for the day. This is keeping you busy during your fasting period.

As time progresses throughout the day, you find yourself working intently, and all of a sudden, your alarm informs you that it is time to eat. Strangely enough, you did not notice you were hungry because you were focused on your work. This is a benefit of being busy; we often forget to eat. So now it's 10 am, and you are eating your first meal of the day. This can consist of any keto-friendly breakfast or lunch options. The thing about Intermittent Fasting with the Keto diet is that you only want to eat about 400 calories in the 1st and 2nd meal of the day. You want to save the bulk of your caloric value until the 3rd meal of the day. So, while at work, you are eating only about 800 calories, and your third meal of the day should be consumed shortly after you get home from work. This will leave you full and satisfied until you start all over again the next day.

This is a simple example of how you can incorporate the Intermittent Fasting and Keto Diet into your day. There are other ways to do this without having to bring food with you every day. However, this was just one example. The important thing to remember when doing the Intermittent Fasting and Keto diet is that you should eat low-carb, high-fat, and moderate protein.

How can you incorporate Intermittent Fasting and the Keto diet into your meal planning?

Meal planning is something that is gaining great popularity with housewives and health advocates alike. When we plan our meals for the week, it takes the guesswork out of what to eat to stay on our healthy diet plan. Incorporating the Intermittent Fasting and Keto diet into your meal plans will be easy if you have already been planning meal plans. If not, then there will be a learning curve, but it can be a simple process by following a few simple rules.

1. Remember that you are fasting during the morning so anything you plan has to be an appropriate meal for breakfast, lunch, or brunch.

2. Remember that you are getting all of your caloric intake within 3 meals so make the best of your food options and caloric breakdown.

3. Do not overindulge in your favorite healthy options. Just because you love it doesn't mean you won't tire of it.

4. Break your caloric intake down into 400 per the first two meals and 800 for the last one. Making sure to put the bulk of your caloric value in your 3rd meal of the day.

5. Give yourself a break, and don't expect perfection right away. It will take some adjusting, and eventually, you will work out a plan that works for you every time.

6. Make a calendar that represents each day of the week where you can either place images of the meals you will be cooking or write into the spaces what meal is for each day so you are prepared a week in advance.

7. Make sure you make a grocery list of just the ingredients you will need and only purchase those ingredients. This will limit any snacking and cravings.

8. Schedule your meals by the day and time you are going to eat them. This will help you have a plan that is specific.

9. Have fun. What is meal prep without fun?

How to fit this diet into your lifestyle and adjust it to fit your health goals

Brief Overview of this chapter

- In this chapter, we discussed how you can incorporate exercise into the Intermittent Fasting and Keto diet and how it will help you. We also talked about changes to the diet that must be made if you do incorporate exercise into your plan.

- Next, we discussed incorporating the Intermittent Fasting and Keto diet into your work lifestyle as well as how you can incorporate it into your meal prep planning.

Chapter 7:
Tips and tricks to make this diet sustainable for everyday life

Why people tend to fail with this diet

Oftentimes, people fail with this diet because they try to rush the results, and instead of following the procedure, they derail the whole process. If you jump straight into a 24-hour fasting or a period of time that is too long for you, then you will find that it is harder to succeed due to the adjustment time that your body needs.

To start an Intermittent Fasting and Keto diet, you should take things slowly and make sure you are not getting ahead of yourself.

Supplements that you can use while on this diet

Because your body is being metabolically changed into ketosis, you will need to ensure that you have the proper supplements to keep your body from being too stressed or being damaged. During ketosis, your gallbladder and your liver are releasing fats that have been stored; they then turn them into ketones. This starts the process of ketosis which is a huge change in the way your body works. It will be an adjustment period that could be painful while you wait for your body to settle. Supplements support you through this change with little to no pain.

Although most people do not require supplements while going into ketosis, it is a very helpful resource. Supplements can help with many things during ketosis.

1. They can reduce uncomfortable symptoms of the Keto flu. We discussed the Keto flu earlier in this book so we will just touch lightly on this part. The Keto flu can be quite painful so supplements can help with this transition.

2. With supplements, you can fill in the nutritional gaps that you are experiencing from the Keto diet.

3. They also help to enhance or maximize your Keto results. This can manifest in an increase in energy levels and a faster weight loss.

4. When you use supplements during the transformation of ketosis, you will be a better version of yourself.

There are 9 Keto supplements that can help you.

1. Electrolytes help us replace potassium, magnesium, sodium, and calcium. These generally come from foods that we would usually be eating. However, on the Keto diet, we are no longer eating those foods. This can cause a decrease in these nutrients, and this can result in a decrease of nerve and muscle function. Due to the Keto diet, our kidneys begin dumping excess water, excreting sodium, and losing electrolytes. Such low levels can lead to headaches, constipation, fatigue, and something called the Keto flu which we have already discussed. Here are the four biggest electrolytes to be aware of:

- Sodium

- Magnesium

- Potassium

- Calcium

2. Vitamin D, which acts as both a nutrient and a hormone, can be lost during the Keto diet. Many of our foods are fortified with vitamin D. You can get it from sun exposure but only in super sunny places. The downside is that extended sun exposure can be the leading cause of skin cancer. Vitamin D is a nutrient that helps your body absorb magnesium, calcium, and other minerals. These are necessary for strength maintenance and muscle growth as well as bone density, a healthy cardiovascular system, immune system support, and testosterone levels that are healthy. Even though we need all the functions, most Americans are low in Vitamin D. With the Keto diet, you could be at even greater risk.

3. MCT which is medium chain triglycerides. They are a form of fat the body uses for energy right away instead of placing the fat in storage. The MCT helps produce ketones. Although ketones are a more efficient energy source than glucose, it is not the easiest process to go into ketosis. By using a supplement of MCT, you can immediately start placing your body into ketosis.

4. Fish oil is great for heart and brain functions. Your body needs 3 forms of Omega-3 fatty acids: DHA, ALA, EPA. This supplement can provide the body with EPA and DHA. However, to get the ALA, we have to eat plant-based foods like walnuts, chia seeds, and vegetable oils. Your body is designed to convert ALA to EPA and DHA. However, it is a very low conversion ratio. Even though the Keto diet is high in Omega-3s, it is also high in Omega-6s which cause inflammation when eaten in excessive amounts. You should eat a ration of 1:1 for omega-3s and omega-6s. Omega-3s are a crucial supplement for brain function as well as heart function.

5. Exogenous ketones are great for ketosis anytime. This is an external supplement of ketones. It can help you get into a ketosis state faster and provides you with additional energy. They are a great supplement to the keto diet.

6. Keto greens are beneficial for a full nutritional support. Drinking a high-quality greens powder will be more beneficial in the long run. It is a great way to cover all of your supplemental needs. There are four different blends that it contains:

    •   Greens blend

    •   Antioxidant blend

    •   Berry blend

- Absorption blend

- Place one scoop in your favorite drink about three times a day.

Brief Overview of this Chapter

- *In this chapter, we discussed why people tend to fail on the Intermittent Fasting and Keto diet and how they can change it.*

- *We talked about supplements that can be used with the Intermittent Fasting and Keto diet and why you would need them.*

Conclusion

Thank you for making it through to the end of *Intermittent Fasting and the Keto Diet*. Let's hope it was informative and able to provide you with all of the tools you need to achieve your goals, whatever they may be.

The next step is to decide how you want to start your journey with Intermittent Fasting and the Keto diet. Make sure you talk with your healthcare professional, and if they agree it is a great fit for you, then plan your fasting period and start slowly decreasing your eating times. It is always best to start slowly with anything new. So remember to succeed at anything, you need to be patient and take it one step at a time. We have included recipes in this book for you to use to get started with the Keto diet. As advised in this book, it is best to get a few weeks into ketosis before you start the Intermittent Fasting portion of this diet plan. However, once you start the fasting, you should see an increase in your Ketosis process. This allows you to go into ketosis much faster. There are also detailed descriptions of supplements that you can take to help you through the Keto diet. Be aware that you will possibly need to pick up some extras supplements if you are finding it hard to maintain your nutritional values. As with any new diet plan, exercise is key to staying in shape so check out the chapter on exercise and incorporate some movement into your day.

Finally, if you found this book useful in any way, a review on Amazon is always appreciated!

Printed in Great Britain
by Amazon

21783291R00079